Finals in Surgery

D0182822

Commissioning Editor: Laurence Hunter
Development Editor: Barbara Simmons
Project Manager: Jess Thompson
Design Direction: Erik Bigland
Cartoons: Charles Simpson
Illustrator: Oxford Illustrators

Finals in Surgery

A Guide to Success in Clinical Surgery

THIRD EDITION

Alastair M. Thompson

ALCM, BSc(Hons), MBChB, MD, FRCSEd(Gen)
Professor of Surgical Oncology, Department of Surgery and Molecular
Oncology, Ninewells Hospital and Medical School, Dundee, UK

Kenneth G. M. Park

MD, FRCSEd
Consultant Surgeon, Aberdeen Royal Infirmary, Aberdeen, UK

ELSEVIER
CHURCHILL
LIVINGSTONE

Edinburgh   London   New York   Oxford   Philadelphia   St Louis   Sydney   Toronto   2008

CHURCHILL
LIVINGSTONE
ELSEVIER

An imprint of Elsevier Limited

© Pearson Professional Limited 1997
© Harcourt Publishers Limited 2001
© 2008, Elsevier Limited. All rights reserved.

First edition 1997
Second edition 2001
Third edition 2008

ISBN-13: 978-0-443-10406-0

British Library Cataloguing in Publication Data
A catalogue record for this book is available from the British Library

Library of Congress Cataloging in Publication Data
A catalog record for this book is available from the Library of Congress

Note
Neither the Publisher nor the authors assume any responsibility for any loss or injury and/or damage to persons or property arising out of or related to any use of the material contained in this book. It is the responsibility of the treating practitioner, relying on independent expertise and knowledge of the patient, to determine the best treatment and method of application for the patient.

The Publisher

ELSEVIER   your source for books,
journals and multimedia
in the health sciences

www.elsevierhealth.com

Working together to grow
libraries in developing countries

www.elsevier.com | www.bookaid.org | www.sabre.org

ELSEVIER   BOOK AID
International   Sabre Foundation

The
publisher's
policy is to use
paper manufactured
from sustainable forests

Printed in China

Contents

Preface

This book has been written to help you pass your surgical finals and should help postgraduate students revise for membership or fellowship of a College of Surgeons. Although not intended as a complete textbook of surgery, it should guide you as to what to expect in surgical finals, assist in your revision and suggest ways of answering common questions. Although much of the book concentrates on traditional long and short cases, the same approach is very effective in Objective Structured Clinical Examinations (OSCEs), and there is a section on topics that may come up in any part of an exam.

In this edition, clinical photographs and diagrams of anatomical or pathological features have been added, the majority from *General Surgical Anatomy and Examination*, IE by Alastair M. Thompson, published by Elsevier. These should help further when you meet patients with the conditions illustrated.

At the end of each chapter, there are key questions to give you practice with examiners' favourites. These also act as revision questions for the chapter – try them out with your colleagues before the exam.

We hope that you will find this book helps you to prepare for surgical examinations and that some of the concepts may be useful in your future clinical practice.

AMT
KGMP
2007

Acknowledgements

This book has been inspired by the teaching of Alastair Munro, Surgeon, Inverness, Andrew Kerr, Anatomist, Edinburgh, and comments from many undergraduate and postgraduate students of surgery worldwide.

We are particularly indebted to colleagues in Dundee (Robert Wood, David Smith, Rodney Mountain, Robert Steele and Peter Stonebridge), Glasgow (Laura Wilkinson), Birmingham (Steve Wigmore) and Aberdeen (Fenton Wallis) for contributions, criticisms and support.

Many patients, the Medical Media Department in Dundee, and Barbara Simmons and Laurence Hunter at Elsevier have made this book possible and to them we are most grateful.

Symbols used in this book

Concentrate your efforts on knowing about the common conditions:

   ★ indicates cases that frequently crop up in surgical examinations

  ★★ indicates cases that are less common

★★★ indicates more complicated cases that occur only rarely

  1 indicates an abnormality on the clinical picture

  ② indicates a normal structure on the clinical picture

1

General principles

THE EXAM IN GENERAL

Depending on whether or not you want to be a surgeon, surgery represents either the pinnacle of human achievement or a specialty populated by sociopaths of varying degrees of adaptation. In either case, surgical examinations are a hurdle that must be overcome.

The aims of this book are to describe a simple and logical approach to surgical examinations and to give examples of common topics and questions to help you to overcome this hurdle. Some of the content may also be useful after you have graduated. However, this book is intended not as a textbook of surgery, but as a helping hand during the few weeks before finals.

WHAT IS EXPECTED OF YOU?

During clinical examinations, it is important to realize that it is not just factual knowledge that is required. The examiners will be assessing your:

- communication skills and attitude to patients
- ability to take a history
- examination technique
- presentation skills
- core knowledge
- deductive reasoning.

During different sections of your exam more emphasis is placed on certain aspects of surgery; in the clinicals the emphasis is quite rightly on clinical skills. Core knowledge is more appropriately tested in your written papers.

PREPARATION FOR THE EXAM

There may be times when you think that you will never know enough to pass an exam (in whatever subject), but fortunately most students are wrong in this respect! Good preparation can minimize the stress caused by finals. A reasonable amount of effort, inspiring teaching, reliable books, consistent attendance at lectures, seminars and tutorials, and above all exposure to real patients with real problems throughout the undergraduate teaching programme will help you to get through finals.

For textbooks in surgery, small is beautiful, although a text that is too small may not cover the subject adequately for the purpose of passing finals. Select undergraduate textbooks that you find readable: choose a book on clinical examination/surgical signs and find another book aimed at getting you through the exam (if you're reading this, you have made a good choice!).

A good way of learning is to browse through your books, looking up topics that you have covered that day on the ward or in teaching sessions. This helps most people to consolidate information, so that key concepts and principles are retained for much longer than when topics or lists are memorized in isolation. Note down any points that you don't really understand and raise them with your fellow students (who are probably puzzled by the same things) and with your teachers on the surgical wards (who may also have to think quite hard). It is better to understand principles on which you can later hang a few facts than to memorize a few facts out of context. This philosophy underlies the increasing emphasis on problem-based learning as opposed to the retention of vast amounts of information, most of which will be forgotten within hours of completing an exam.

During the few days before your exams, ensure that you are familiar with the topics that are usually covered. Being an expert on heart transplantation is of no advantage if you know little about hip fractures, colorectal cancer or thyroid swellings: the first will not come up in finals, but the other three topics almost certainly will. If you have a few minutes to spare (unlikely though this may seem), looking through the tables and illustrations in the books that you have used is well worthwhile.

Finally, getting a good night's sleep before the exam is more valuable than trying to cram a few extra facts into a tired, caffeine-saturated brain. An alert candidate with a little knowledge is likely to think more clearly, answer questions more lucidly and fare better in the exam than a sleep-deprived swot. Remember that the examiners are assessing you and your ability to think logically – this is more likely to impress than one or two extra facts. Sleep deprivation is not a compulsory part of the undergraduate curriculum and is becoming less and less common even for junior hospital doctors.

Failure in surgical finals is guaranteed if you arrive after the exam has finished. Make sure that you know where (not just which hospital, but which ward) and when the exam will take place. Set out in good time: it is better to arrive an hour early and approach the exam outwardly composed than to worry that the traffic is making you late and arrive as a ruffled sweaty heap with your mind in a turmoil. If it looks as if you are going to be late, try to phone; if you are late, make apologies: in some situations, the examiners may try to accommodate you.

PERSONAL PRESENTATION (Fig. 1.1)

In most clinical exams, including surgical ones, tradition dictates that you dress smartly but comfortably and that you present yourself in a recently washed state. Dirty fingernails and hands or an untamed head or face of hair is not likely to appeal to either the examiners or the patients. Although a T-shirt and shorts may seem right on a hot day, the jacket and tie or 'sensible' blouse and skirt are more likely to get the examiners and patients looking upon you with confidence as a future doctor. This is not an occasion for experimenting with the latest fad in fashion! Some institutions suggest a white coat as standard attire in the exam, but the above points still apply. Whether you wear normal clothing or a white coat, a clear name badge can be helpful in identifying yourself to the examiners and patients.

EQUIPMENT (Fig. 1.1)

For a surgical exam you do not need to appear laden with heavy-duty medical equipment, prepared for every eventuality. The key essentials for a basic surgical exam are your eyes, ears, hands and brain. To complement these, you need a watch, a stethoscope, a measuring tape, a pen torch, and a pen and paper. Anything else that you need should be provided, including a tendon hammer, a tuning fork, cotton wool, disposable needles, an ophthalmoscope, a blood pressure cuff, urine testing sticks, a tourniquet and gloves.

Fig. 1.1 Exam candidates should be presentable and carry only the essentials for surgical finals.

EXAMINERS

Examiners come in a variety of shapes, sizes and ages and with a range of countenances. They usually hunt in pairs so as to outnumber the candidate (Fig. 1.2)! One may be an 'internal' examiner, from the institution running the exam, and the other an 'external' examiner from St Elsewhere. Although this pairing can make them seem pretty intimidating, it is really to ensure fair play. Examiners should introduce themselves to you, and may already know something about the patients whom you see. If one examiner knows you (from your time on the wards or because you beat him or her in the annual medical school golf competition), he or she may opt to swap places with a colleague or simply listen.

Fig. 1.2 Examiners usually hunt in pairs: the good guy and the bad guy.

Unfortunately, even if you are to be assessed by an examiner whom you feel may not ensure fair play, it may not be possible to swap with another candidate: check with the person running the exam.

The examiners should mark you according to a schedule, which may be divided into categories such as: approach to the patient; history-taking; clinical examination of the patient; presentational skills; and ability to interpret findings and answer questions.

The examiners will confer with each other after you have left, and will decide what mark to award you for that component of the exam. The various marks you receive will be collated, and borderline candidates (for distinction or pass/fail) may undergo further assessment.

KEY POINTS

- Prepare for the exam in good time
- Try to grasp the concepts and principles onto which you can hang facts
- Use books to consolidate information on patients you have seen or topics you have discussed
- Approach the exam rested, smartly dressed and outwardly cool, calm and collected
- Take to the exam a watch, stethoscope, tape, torch, pen and paper
- Remember examiners generally want you to get through the exam

THE EXAM IN DETAIL

Most patients involved in the clinical exams are either patients in the wards at the time of the exam (preoperative patients, patients admitted for investigation or, occasionally, postoperative patients) or outpatients who have been brought to the hospital to help with the exam (often having a hernia, varicose veins, orthopaedic problems or a skin lesion).

EXAMINATION OF THE PATIENT

Before examining a patient, it is wise formally to introduce yourself (you may have been told the patient's name, but he or she probably does not know yours), and to establish contact with the patient by shaking hands. This usually gets the patient on your side and shows that you too are human (if a little frightened), and so gets the exam off to a good start. Beware the rare patient who has a painful hand (perhaps with a drip in place) or who has a paralysed right upper limb, an amputation or a congenital limb deformity: you may find yourself shaking the left, instead of the right, hand! A chaperone is advisable, particularly for male students or doctors examining a female patient, and is essential for breast, rectal or gynaecological examination.

It is traditional to stand at the patient's right-hand side, particularly if you are going to examine the chest or abdomen. This has the advantage of familiarity: if you always approach and examine the patient in the same way, you will have developed a sense of security before your exam. Also, you are much more likely to detect abnormalities.

Remember to look for clues, particularly in the traditional long case, during which you are likely to be left with the patient for between 20 minutes and an hour. TPR (temperature/pulse/blood pressure/respiratory rate) charts may show pyrexia or a change in pulse or blood pressure over time. Drug charts may hint at not only the disease(s) that the patient has but also their investigation and management. Radiographs are sometimes left with the patient and can give helpful hints as to how the patient has been investigated (look at the envelope containing the radiographs) and even indicate the diagnosis. Some patients have been involved in surgical finals before, and if you strike it lucky with a cooperative patient who knows a lot about his or her condition, the exam can become almost enjoyable. Even so, don't forget to cover the basics.

For both undergraduate and postgraduate clinical examinations, four formats may be used: the long case, short cases, orals and Objective

Structured Clinical Examinations (OSCEs). Ensure that you are familiar with the structure of the examinations that you are about to sit.

LONG CASE

The traditional surgical long case usually involves the candidate being allocated a patient. You are required to take a history and examine the patient and then present the case, suggest how to investigate the patient and discuss the surgical and non-surgical management. In the long case you will be assessed initially on your presentation skills, and thereafter on your ability to think logically about possible diagnoses, appropriate investigations and management.

The secret to performing well in a long case is to take an accurate history with sufficient relevant details and to examine the patient appropriately, paying particular attention to the condition(s) from which the patient suffers. Make short notes as you go, but don't waste time scripting a beautifully written history: the emphasis of the exam is on oral communication of your history taking and on your clinical examination skills. Having noted the main findings of the history and examination, write down the investigations that you would order, then list the treatment options. Beware: patients selected for long cases often suffer from more than one condition (e.g. breast cancer, ischaemic heart disease and osteoarthritis), so you have to remember to outline the relevant findings, investigations and treatments for each condition and indicate how they are interrelated.

Try to set aside 5 minutes before the examiners pounce, so that you can organize your thoughts and present them coherently.

The general scheme for a long case, which can be truncated for short cases or OSCEs, is shown in Table 1.1. You should adapt this to suit you and should practise the scheme many times before the exam.

Table 1.1 Approach to the patient		
Introduction	Inspection	Investigation
Permission	Palpation	Diagnosis
History	Percussion	Treatment
Exposure	Auscultation	
Position		

HISTORY

Write down key words and phrases as you go:

- Name and age of patient
- Problem(s)/presenting symptom(s)
- Systematic enquiry for each problematic system
- Past medical/surgical history
- Drug history/allergies/alcohol/smoking
- Social history, including home circumstances and support
- Occupation
- Family history
- Systematic enquiry for systems not already covered.

Unfortunately not all patients are cooperative (Fig. 1.3): sometimes communication is difficult (e.g. the hearing-impaired patient who has lost his teeth, is very talkative, and speaks with a curious accent that you can't quite understand); or the patient doesn't really want to participate in the exam (just like you) and takes it out on you. Occasionally, a patient may become unwell during the long case: you should alert the exam supervisor. Nursing staff can be particularly helpful,

Fig. 1.3 Patients can be helpful or, like you, may not really want to participate in the exam.

especially in an emergency. The patient may, however, understand the exam situation and spill the beans freely to you (including all the investigations and treatments to date if you're lucky). Even so, ensure that you have asked all the relevant questions: it is all too easy to accept at face value all that is volunteered and miss out on some essential points. For example, a patient who tells you his gallstones were revealed by ultrasound scanning and that he has had pancreatitis still needs to be asked about alcohol consumption.

There are patients with complex histories who may happily fill an hour by just giving you their life story. With practice (so do not attempt it for the first time in the exam) it is possible to obtain part of the patient's history while you perform the physical examination: you may see this being done in outpatient clinics or on ward rounds.

CLINICAL EXAMINATION

Note abnormal findings (Fig. 1.4):

- General features (jaundice, anaemia, cyanosis, clubbing, oedema, lymphadenopathy, cachexia, etc.)
- Head and neck examination
- Cardiovascular system
- Respiratory system
- Breast examination
- Abdominal examination (no rectal or vaginal examination in the exam)
- Limb and back examination
- Neurological examination (central and peripheral).

One way to approach the examination in a long case is illustrated in Fig. 1.4. As you proceed through the patient's examination, note down positive and important findings.

SUMMARY OF PATIENT

- Introduction (e.g. 'Mr John Knox, a 72-year-old former preacher . . .')
- Problems (e.g. '. . . who presents with . . . [one sentence]')
- Main findings ('On examination . . . [one or two sentences]').

DIFFERENTIAL DIAGNOSIS

- Principal problems
- Other problem(s).

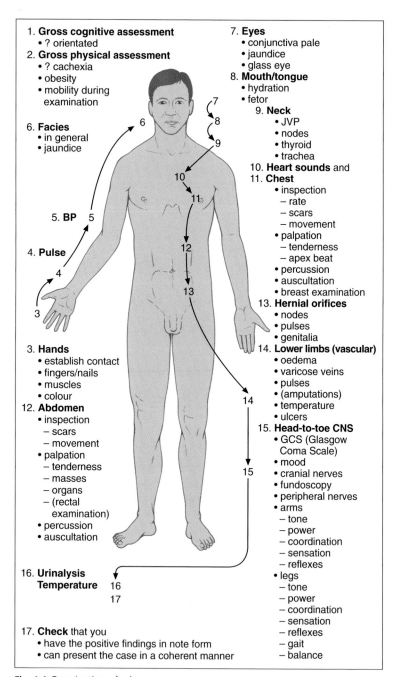

1. **Gross cognitive assessment**
   • ? orientated
2. **Gross physical assessment**
   • ? cachexia
   • obesity
   • mobility during examination

6. **Facies**
   • in general
   • jaundice

5. **BP** 5

4. **Pulse**

3. **Hands**
   • establish contact
   • fingers/nails
   • muscles
   • colour
12. **Abdomen**
   • inspection
     − scars
     − movement
   • palpation
     − tenderness
     − masses
     − organs
     − (rectal examination)
   • percussion
   • auscultation

16. **Urinalysis**
    Temperature 16
                     17

17. **Check** that you
    • have the positive findings in note form
    • can present the case in a coherent manner

7. **Eyes**
   • conjunctiva pale
   • jaundice
   • glass eye
8. **Mouth/tongue**
   • hydration
   • fetor
9. **Neck**
   • JVP
   • nodes
   • thyroid
   • trachea
10. **Heart sounds** and
11. **Chest**
   • inspection
     − rate
     − scars
     − movement
   • palpation
     − tenderness
     − apex beat
   • percussion
   • auscultation
   • breast examination
13. **Hernial orifices**
   • nodes
   • pulses
   • genitalia
14. **Lower limbs (vascular)**
   • oedema
   • varicose veins
   • pulses
   • (amputations)
   • temperature
   • ulcers
15. **Head-to-toe CNS**
   • GCS (Glasgow Coma Scale)
   • mood
   • cranial nerves
   • fundoscopy
   • peripheral nerves
   • arms
     − tone
     − power
     − coordination
     − sensation
     − reflexes
   • legs
     − tone
     − power
     − coordination
     − sensation
     − reflexes
     − gait
     − balance

Fig. 1.4 Examination of a long case.

INVESTIGATIONS

The emphasis, when discussing investigations, must be on:

1. Starting with the simple, non-invasive tests – building on these accordingly.
2. Investigations appropriate to the patient's condition.

Choose from the following list the appropriate tests for the patient whom you have seen:

- Urine dipstick test:
  - biochemistry/microbiology
  - pregnancy test
- Faeces:
  - occult blood
  - microbiology
  - tests of gastrointestinal function
- Blood tests, including:
  - haematology, coagulation
  - biochemistry
  - microbiology
  - immunology
  - blood transfusion
  - hormone levels
- Cardiology:
  - ECG
  - echocardiography
- Radiology:
  - skull and cervical spine radiograph
  - chest radiograph
  - abdominal/pelvic radiograph
  - limb radiograph
  - contrast studies of:
    - gastrointestinal tract
    - vascular tree
    - urological system
  - ultrasound and Doppler scanning
  - computed tomography
  - magnetic resonance imaging
  - radionuclide imaging
- Surgical studies:
  - upper endoscopy
  - endoscopic retrograde cholangiopancreatography (ERCP)

- proctoscopy
- rigid sigmoidoscopy
- flexible sigmoidoscopy/colonoscopy
- Physiological studies:
  - upper gastrointestinal tract
  - lower gastrointestinal tract
  - urinary system
  - nervous system
- Pathology:
  - cytology
  - biopsy.

For example, a patient with jaundice should have urinalysis, faecal occult blood testing, haematology, coagulation and biochemistry, followed by ultrasound before proceeding to ERCP.

MANAGEMENT

- Conservative measures (modify diet, stop smoking, etc.)
- Medical therapy (fluids, analgesia, etc.)
- Chemotherapy
- Radiotherapy
- Surgery.

Approach to a long case

For a long case, allow yourself approximately the times shown in Table 1.2.

Obviously, there is a lot of similarity between approaching a long case in surgical exams and approaching one in medical exams. Some

Table 1.2 Use of time in a long case		
Length of case	1 hour	30 min
History	20 min	10 min
Examination	20 min	10 min
Summary/differential diagnosis	5 min	3 min
Investigations/plan management	5 min	3 min
Organize/go over presentation/think through some questions	10 min	4 min

medical schools combine the two and give you a single long case, usually cunningly selecting a patient with both medical and surgical problems.

Practise seeing patients under simulated exam conditions in the lead-up to your exam, recording the information listed above and then presenting the patient to a fellow student or qualified doctor. A competently conducted history and examination, thoughtfully presented to your examiners, will give you the best possible basis on which to succeed in finals.

PRESENTATION

The oral presentation about the patient whom you have just seen is something that becomes easier with practice. Aim to present the exam patient in the way that you have previously presented patients to your fellow students and teachers. Speak slowly and clearly, and use medical terminology precisely, so that the examiners can follow you. Emphasize the positive points and, if there are a number of problems or disease processes, deal with these one at a time. Avoid reeling off a list of negative findings: carefully chosen phrases such as 'on systematic enquiry, there were no abnormal genitourinary or neurological symptoms' or 'on examination, the cardiovascular and respiratory systems were otherwise normal' can be used to good effect.

Don't be put off by apparent inattention on the part of your examiners – they may still be listening carefully. Examiners can be quite irritating and may interrupt your masterful presentation to ask further questions. They may simply want to clarify a point. Alternatively, they may launch into questioning because it has become clear to them that you have no idea about the patient (unlikely), or because you have convinced them that your history/examination technique is adequate and they can't wait to start quizzing your finely tuned, razor-sharp mind! Occasionally, you may have identified things in the history or examination that the examiners hadn't spotted or you may have missed an important feature: the examiners will then feel entitled to take you back to review the patient. Even if you have got something wrong, the situation may be retrieved by staying outwardly calm, doing as the examiners ask, admitting your mistake and changing your answer if necessary.

SHORT CASE

In many ways, short cases are a rehearsal for your professional life as a hospital doctor in outpatient or accident and emergency departments, or for general practice surgeries. One excellent way to prepare for short cases is to attend surgical outpatient clinics. This will give you practice, sometimes under the eyes of your future examiners, at taking a concise history (with perhaps three key open-ended questions), at examining the relevant systems, speedily but accurately, and at establishing the symptoms, signs and underlying condition(s). The emphasis in short cases is on how you interrogate a patient, given a starting point, or how you examine a system. The more you have practised examining and are familiar with a system of examination, the more relaxed you will seem and the better you will perform. You will then come to your finals in the knowledge that you can confidently and competently address most of the short case topics likely to come up in the exam.

As mentioned already, it is worthwhile introducing yourself to the patient and establishing contact by shaking hands. In the few seconds that this takes you may get some clues about the condition(s) from which the patient suffers, e.g. a walking stick or obvious musculoskeletal deformities may suggest that the patient has had orthopaedic treatment for arthritis.

You may be asked to take a brief history (e.g. by asking 'What are the main problems that have brought you to the hospital?') or simply to examine the patient. Listen carefully to what your examiner asks.

CLINICAL EXAMINATION

Examination should follow the scheme:

- Exposure/position
- Inspection
- Palpation
- Percussion
- Auscultation.

This is modified for orthopaedic examinations to:

- Exposure/position
- Look
- Feel
- Move.

Exposure/position means that you need to ensure that clothing has been removed from the part of the body that you are about to inspect. Both limbs should be exposed in the case of a limb problem (without socks remaining to hide something relevant), the abdomen should be exposed from nipple to groin and, for the examination of the head and neck, the shirt should be removed, and not just the collar loosened, to allow adequate visualization of the neck. The patient should be positioned so that you can examine the appropriate area and so that he or she is comfortable (and hence remains cooperative). Before palpation, always ask if there is any tenderness. Apparently comfortable patients can turn you into a nervous wreck if you grasp a tender, rheumatoid limb.

Approach to a short case

Pay attention to what the examiner actually asks you. Compare 'Describe this skin lesion' (a specific question) with 'Examine this patient's groin': in the latter, there may be any number of problems, and you need to go through the examination scheme for the groin carefully. To ensure that the examiners appreciate what you are demonstrating, you may wish to talk your way through a short case. An examiner may interrupt your examination and ask you about your findings so far and how you would proceed. Alternatively, an examiner may direct you to repeat or perform a particular manoeuvre to get you to elicit a specific sign.

While you examine a patient, be alert for clues that may suggest the diagnosis (e.g. a glass of water to assist swallowing during examination of the thyroid). It is worthwhile trying to think through some of the things that you may be asked about, e.g. a palpable thyroid lump may prompt you to think of the symptoms and signs of hyperthyroidism, or finger clubbing may alert you to recall the various possible causes of clubbing. This will give you the edge when the examiner asks those same questions!

ORAL EXAMS

Most examiners will ask questions (and expect answers!) stemming from your presentation of the long case or as part of the short cases, but in some medical schools there are separate face-to-face question-and-answer sessions, usually lasting 5–20 minutes. Sometimes, the oral exam can cover anaesthetics, microbiology relevant to surgery, laboratory investigations (biochemistry, haematology) or pathology.

As for the clinical exam, an appropriate standard of dress and degree of decorum are required for oral (viva voce) exams. Before, during and after this part of an exam, you may feel nervous, frightened, intimidated and completely ignorant of all things surgical, and wish that a hole in the ground would swallow you up. This is very common! Most examiners understand this, and should put you at your ease by starting off with a simple question.

The golden rules for oral examinations are to wait for the examiner to finish asking the question, think briefly before you open your mouth and then speak clearly. Start with general features and then go on to specific points, and mention common conditions before rarities. Giving scorpion stings as a cause of pancreatitis suggests that you are clueless about its common causes (alcohol and gallstones), not that you are well read. If you know a lot about the topic about which you have been asked, keep talking – the examiner will interrupt you soon enough.

When asked about the management of a particular condition, it is worthwhile starting with 'Having taken a history and examined the patient . . .'. If asked about the treatment of a patient, start with 'Having taken a history, examined and appropriately investigated this man with colonic carcinoma . . .'.

If an examiner challenges something that you have said, either stick to your statement ('Yes, femoral hernias are more common in women than in men') or correct the error that you may have made ('I should have said femoral hernias are more common in women than in men, not the other way round'). Sometimes examiners may say that you are wrong: it is better to accept their judgement (whatever you may secretly think!) and move on to the next topic than to enter into an argument that you cannot win, even if you are right. In effect, the examiners make the rules, field the opposing team and act as referee. If the questions get difficult, this usually means that you are doing well, so don't be discouraged. The examiners may even start to impart some of their own wisdom to you!

When answering the questions, try to structure your answers as follows:

- History (symptoms)
- Examination (signs, including urinalysis)
- Investigations (blood, radiology, microbiology, pathology, special tests such as endoscopy)
- Diagnosis
- Management/treatment (conservative, medical, chemotherapy, radiotherapy or surgical).

Even if you know little about the topic in question, by answering in this structured way you may be able to scrape together enough information to satisfy the examiners. The sequence of history (symptoms), examination (signs), investigations, diagnosis and management/treatment forms the basic structure not only for examinations but also for medical practice in real life in outpatient clinics, A&Es and general practice surgeries. So this simple approach to clinical problems (not just in surgery) can help get you through life as a medical graduate as well as through exams.

OBJECTIVE STRUCTURED CLINICAL EXAMINATIONS

An OSCE is, as the name suggests, designed to assess individual students objectively with structured questions. By using a predetermined, structured, marking regime and patients (or actors) who have known clinical histories and examination findings, the OSCE should standardize what students are asked and the way in which they are marked, cutting out the subjective and variable standards of conventional exams. An OSCE exam may comprise several different topics with the candidates moving between individual stations, e.g. there may be ten stations, two on history taking (jaundiced patient, change in bowel habit), three on clinical examination (chest, lower limb, abdomen), three on investigations (an abdominal film, some blood results, urine test), one on communication skills and one on cardiopulmonary resuscitation. Thus an OSCE-style examination may test many of the skills and techniques outlined earlier in this chapter that you would apply to traditional long case/short case/oral examinations.

In the OSCE you may be asked to take a relevant history, with the examiner marking your questions relating to the history and/or investigations and treatment of the patient's condition. You are thus being tested on how good your history-taking skills are against the same marking schedule that is used for the other candidates. Alternatively, you may be asked to 'examine the abdomen of this man who presented with . . .'. Marks are allocated for elements of the examination technique correctly performed, positive clinical findings noted, and answers to questions about investigations and treatment. Similarly you may be asked to inspect a limb for signs of acute ischaemia. As you state the features that you find, the examiner will award the marks indicated on the marking schedule for: pale (1); pulseless (1); painful (1); paraesthesia (1); and perishingly cold (1); the maximum score is 5 marks. There may be questions on the causes of the ischaemia, complications and/or the possible treatments: conservative measures (stop smoking, increase exercise) (2); medical therapy (1); surgical therapy (angioplasty, arterial reconstruction, amputation) (3).

There should, theoretically, be no subjective component of the marking schedule – eliminating the variations in the questions that the examiners ask and the level of knowledge that they expect, and thereby making it a fairer exam. However, time constraints and examiner boredom limit the use of OSCEs in some medical schools.

KEY POINTS

- Practice is the best way to success in clinical examinations
- Always introduce yourself to the patient and wash your hands
- Look for clues (e.g. walking stick, charts, radiographs, glass of water)
- Speak slowly and clearly, and use precise medical terminology
- **Long case**: allocate appropriate lengths of time to:
  - history
  - examination
  - summary/differential diagnosis
  - investigations/plan of management
  - organize/go over presentation/think through some questions
- **Short case**: remember:
  - exposure/position
  - inspection
  - palpation
  - percussion
  - auscultation
- **Short case/oral/OSCE**:
  - listen to the question
  - think
  - answer the question posed.

THE SURGICAL SIEVE

The overall scheme for the assessment and management of any patient can be summarized as follows:

- History (symptoms)
- Examination (signs, including urinalysis)
- Investigations (blood, radiology, microbiology, pathology, special tests such as endoscopy)
- Diagnosis
- Management.

Once you have an idea of the patient's problem(s), it is possible to use the 'surgical sieve' to work out the underlying pathological processes, likely diagnoses and possible management.

The traditional long case is most likely to test your ability to put all of these steps together; however, short cases and OSCEs may test aspects of this, e.g. given that this patient fell on her outstretched arm, can you comment on her radiograph? What is the diagnosis? What are the management options?

CLASSIFICATION OF PROBLEMS

In the case of each problem that you have identified in the history or on examination, consider whether the condition is congenital or acquired and which system(s) it has affected.

Conditions

CONGENITAL

- Inherited
- Developmental

ACQUIRED

- Infective:
  - acute/chronic
  - bacterial/viral/other
- Neoplastic:
  - benign/malignant
  - primary/secondary
- Inflammatory:
  - acute/chronic
  - local/generalized
  - granulomatous/non-granulomatous
- Traumatic:
  - acute/chronic
- Vascular:
  - acute/chronic
  - peripheral/central
  - arterial/venous
- Endocrine:
  - by gland/by mechanism
  - underactive/overactive
- Metabolic:
  - acute/chronic

- Autoimmune:
  - local/generalized
- Degenerative
- Miscellaneous

Systems

- Cardiovascular
- Respiratory
- Gastrointestinal
- Genitourinary
- Central nervous system
- Peripheral nervous system
- Locomotor
- Endocrine
- Skin.

For example, in the case of a patient who presents with a breast lump, the lump may be infective, neoplastic, inflammatory or traumatic, and affecting a hormone-responsive organ. When listing your differential diagnosis, start with the most common cause and work your way down to less common causes.

Another way of classifying conditions, particularly applicable to the mechanical obstruction of a tubular organ (such as the gastrointestinal tract), is based on whether the pathology causing symptoms lies:

- within the lumen
- within the wall
- outside the wall.

For example, a patient with dysphagia caused by obstruction of the oesophagus may have: a bolus obstruction resulting from a food bolus lodging in the lumen of the oesophagus, a malignant stricture in the wall of the oesophagus, or else external compression from a lung tumour.

MANAGEMENT

Having worked out the possible diagnoses, a systematic approach should be used to consider the treatment options for each condition in a particular patient. Try applying this scheme to patients whom you meet on the wards:

- Conservative treatment:
  - prophylactic (e.g. take exercise)
  - stop (e.g. smoking)
  - start (e.g. high–fibre diet)
- Medical treatment:
  - prophylactic (e.g. immunization)
  - curative (e.g. antibiotics)
  - maintenance of function (e.g. digoxin)
- Chemotherapy:
  - adjuvant (e.g. breast or colon cancer)
  - curative (e.g. teratoma)
  - palliative (e.g. liver metastases)
- Radiotherapy:
  - adjuvant (e.g. breast cancer)
  - curative (e.g. basal cell carcinoma)
  - palliative (e.g. bone metastases)
- Surgery:
  - minimally invasive (e.g. endoscopy, interventional radiology)
  - relieving (e.g. abscess)
  - resectional (e.g. appendix, tumour)
  - reconstructive (e.g. arterial graft).

As an example of the use of this systematic approach, consider the case of a patient with splenomegaly and hypersplenism, secondary to idiopathic thrombocytopenic purpura. Conservative measures alone are unlikely to be of benefit, and neither chemotherapy nor radiotherapy is indicated. Medical options include the use of steroids and surgical removal of the spleen (by laparoscopic or by open surgery) is also possible.

COMPLICATIONS

Problems related to surgery and its complications, as well as being classified by condition and system as above, can be classed as one or more of:

- preoperative
- intraoperative
- postoperative.

To complicate matters further, any such complications may:

- be localized or systemic
- be a possible consequence of any operation or be specific to a particular operation
- occur in the short or long term after the surgery.

For example, a patient with a fractured neck of the femur may have cardiorespiratory disease and arrive at hospital with hypothermia (pre-operative, systemic problems that could exist before any operation). After the intraoperative complication of blood loss (localized problem with systemic effects), postoperatively the patient may develop deep venous thrombosis complicated by a pulmonary embolism (localized then systemic problem that may occur after any operation but is more common after hip surgery than after most procedures). Wound infection of the hemiarthroplasty could occur 1 year later (long-term problem specific to joint replacement surgery).

EXAMINERS' FAVOURITES

There are some problems and types of patient that seem to come up time and time again in surgical finals. The top 20 short cases (not in order of importance) probably include:

- abdominal mass
- carpal tunnel syndrome
- basal cell carcinoma
- Dupuytren's contracture
- breast lump
- ganglion
- bunion
- hernia
- ingrown toenail
- pigmented skin lesion
- jaundice
- lipoma
- neck lump
- scrotal swelling
- sebaceous cyst
- stoma
- palpable liver
- thyroid swelling
- peripheral vascular disease
- varicose veins.

The top five long cases are probably:

- abdominal mass
- breast cancer

- gallstone disease
- orthopaedic problem
- peripheral vascular disease.

KEY POINTS

- **Assessment and management** of any patient:
  - history (symptoms)
  - examination (signs)
  - investigations
  - diagnosis
  - management
- **The surgical sieve** identifies conditions as congenital or acquired, in the case of each organ or system affected
- **Management** may be categorized as:
  - conservative
  - medical
  - chemotherapy
  - radiotherapy
  - surgery
- **Complications** may be grouped as:
  - preoperative/intraoperative/postoperative
  - localized/systemic
  - short/long term.

2

Skin, lumps and bumps

Skin lesions, lumps and bumps are very common in short cases in surgical finals. This is partly because such problems are common and can be examined repeatedly by different candidates without up-setting the patient, but also because they test things that you will have seen before and can be used as a talking point for differential diagnoses and treatment. The best way to prepare for skin lesions, lumps and bumps in the exam is to see and examine many such lesions during your time as an undergraduate. However, this is rarely possible and a good second-best alternative is to look up the appearance and features of the common lesions in one of the many good colour atlases of surgery.

As these lesions can be present on almost any part of the body, there is some overlap between the topics covered in this chapter and those in Chapters 3, 5 and 7.

HISTORY

You may not get much chance to take a history from a patient with a skin lesion or lump if the examiners are using the case to carry out a spot check on your observational skills. However, the approximate age of the patient and the location of the lesion will be apparent. If you do get the opportunity to ask anything, key questions should cover the following:

- The duration of the lesion (when it first appeared, whether it has changed since the patient first noticed it)
- Any predisposing events (e.g. sun exposure, trauma, insect bite)
- Whether the lesion is tender
- Whether there has been any change in size, shape or colour (these three points are particularly important if you suspect a melanoma).

Also, ask about the following:

- Any other lesions
- Any associated features (e.g. pain in an inflammatory lymph node; intermittent discharge from a sebaceous cyst; pain of cutaneous nerve distribution)
- What treatment has been suggested or administered.

EXAMINATION

Exposure/position

The examination of a lump or skin lesion, as for any other clinical examination, needs adequate exposure of not just the lesion but the whole region and the regional lymph nodes before progressing to inspection, palpation, percussion and auscultation.

Inspection

During your general approach and introduction to the patient, you should note any general features of disease (jaundice, cachexia, etc.) that you may comment on later. Look at and describe to the examiner the following features of the lesion(s):

- Number (single/multiple)
- Position
- Size (in centimetres: use your measuring tape)
- Shape
- Colour
- Outline of the margin
- Contour of the surface.

If the skin overlying the lesion appears to be intact, observe whether the skin:

- appears tight (thin, shiny)
- appears discoloured (e.g. bluish, erythematous)
- has obvious associated blood vessels.

In the case of an ulcerated lesion, include comments about the following:

- The edge (e.g. sloping, punched out, everted, rolled, undermined)
- The base (e.g. whether there is clean granulation tissue or slough – can you see bone or a tendon?)
- The approximate depth of the ulcer
- The presence or absence of a discharge from the ulcer.

For skin lesions on the limbs, make it obvious to the examiner that you are examining the whole surface of a limb. Ask the patient whether the limb is painful and examine between the toes. Lift up the lower limb to scrutinize its complete circumference, including the heel, and look for other lesions of the skin.

Palpation

Before touching the patient, check whether there is any pain or tenderness and wash your hands.

Feel for a temperature difference between the lesion and the surrounding tissues, traditionally using the back of your fingers. Palpate the lesion very gently to detect any tenderness (tender lumps are unlikely to be in the exam for obvious reasons but, towards the end of an exam, a lump may become tender after examination by several candidates).

Consider the composition of a lump and try to identify whether it is solid or filled with fluid or gas:

- Does it feel hard or soft?
- Is it fluctuant? (The test for fluctuance uses three fingers on a lump that must be at least 2 cm in size.)
- Can the lump be transilluminated? (Use a pen-torch pressed against the skin.)
- Could the lump be vascular?
- Look for pulsatility (which may simply be transmitted).
- Feel whether the lump is expansile.
- Feel for a bruit.
- Assess whether the lesion can be compressed and whether it refills when released (as does a sapheno varix).

The relationship of a skin lesion or subcutaneous lump to the overlying and surrounding tissues may be the key feature in defining the diagnosis. Decide whether a lesion is in the skin itself or in the subcutaneous tissues, and whether a lump is tethered or even fixed to the deeper structures. An assessment can be made of the fixity of the lump to muscles and fascia by asking the patient to contract the underlying muscles. This can also be useful in assessing whether a lump is mobile in all directions or whether mobility is restricted to one direction. Rarely, a lump may result in pain corresponding to the distribution of a local nerve, or even a distal neurological deficit.

Palpation of the regional lymph nodes should not be forgotten: ask the examiner, and then the patient, for permission to examine the regional lymph nodes. For lesions of the lower limb, buttock and perineum, include the inguinal lymph nodes. For lesions of the upper limb, include the epitrochlear, axillary, infraclavicular and supraclavicular nodes. For lesions of the torso, include the groin, axillary, infraclavicular, supraclavicular and cervical nodes, depending on the site of the lesion. For head and neck lesions, remember to examine not just the lymph node most likely to be involved in drainage, but also the other cervical nodes.

Percussion

Percussion may be useful for detecting resonance, if you suspect that there is a gas-filled viscus within a large lump (e.g. a bowel-containing hernia).

Auscultation

Auscultation for a bruit (in the case of a vascular lesion) or bowel sounds should be mentioned to the examiner, and performed, where appropriate.

Further examination

After you have examined a skin lesion or lump, you may be asked whether there are any other things that you would like to do. This usually either means that you have not examined the lesion adequately or is a hint not to forget the regional lymph nodes. If you suspect that the lesion is part of a systemic disease process (such as metastatic malignancy, lymphoma or sarcoidosis), you should suggest that it would be useful to examine for lymphadenopathy elsewhere or to examine organs (e.g. the breast) for the site of a primary tumour or secondary spread (e.g. to the liver).

Summary

Remember the features of a lump that you should comment upon:

- Size
- Shape
- Colour
- Position
- Consistency

- Fixation to skin and/or deeper structures
- Associated features (including regional lymph nodes).

TYPICAL CASES

Some of the lesions you may see are illustrated in Fig. 2.1.

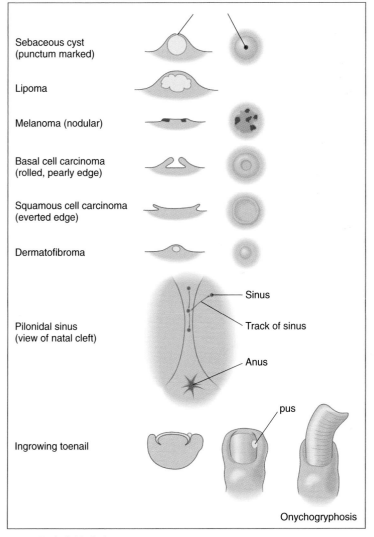

Fig. 2.1 Typical skin lesions.

Sebaceous cyst*

The history is usually of a long-standing lump, and may involve inter-mittent swelling resulting in a cheesy discharge. On examination, a punctum (the opening of the cyst on to the skin surface) is usually visible. The skin is usually immovable over the cyst and tightly adherent to it, because a sebaceous cyst lies within the skin itself.

Sebaceous cysts are frequently found in the scalp, neck, axilla or groin and may be multiple or become infected (Fig. 2.2).

A sebaceous cyst is a popular choice for exams, because it needs to be distinguished from a lipoma (Table 2.1).

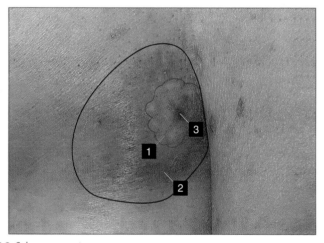

Fig. 2.2 Sebaceous cyst.

1 Sebaceous cyst
2 Erythema
3 Punctum

KEY POINTS

- Punctum
- Arises within the skin

Lipoma*

A lipoma may be solitary, with a long history of slow growth (sometimes to many centimetres in size) or there may be multiple lipomas (often

Table 2.1 Features of common lumps

Lesion	Sebaceous cyst	Lipoma	Lymph node
Size	5 mm–2 cm	1–10+ cm	5 mm–2+ cm
Shape	Spherical	Disc	Bean like
Colour	Skin may be red	Normal skin	Normal skin
Consistency	Soft or hard	Soft/fluctuant	Firm or hard
Position	Scalp/axilla/neck	Trunk/limbs	Neck/axilla/groin
Fixation	To skin	? To muscle	? To muscle
Associated features	Punctum Cheesy exudate		Likely to be multiple

2–4 cm in size). Rarely, lipomas may be tender or compress surrounding structures. A lipoma may appear to be fluctuant because of the semifluid nature of fat at body temperature. It is often lobulated in outline (Fig. 2.3) and ranges in size from 1 to 10 cm. It lies in the subcutaneous tissues, and sometimes passes down through a fascial plane, which results in tethering to the underlying tissues. The skin over a lipoma should be freely mobile and this feature, together with the absence of a punctum, distinguishes it from a sebaceous cyst. A lipoma may recur after resection, and so you may see a scar related to the lump.

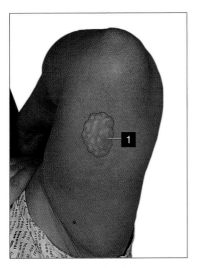

Fig. 2.3 Lipoma.

1 Lipoma

Lymph node*

Single or multiple lymph nodes, in one or several groups, are common short cases because of the frequency of lymphadenopathy in clinical practice. The most important features of lymphadenopathy are the position, number, size, consistency and distribution of the lymph nodes. As a rough guide, soft lymph nodes are probably benign; a rubbery consistency suggests lymphoma and hard lumps suggest metastatic carcinoma. Wherever the nodes are sited, it is imperative that you ask the examiner whether you can examine the region that the nodes drain: axillary nodes drain the upper limb, breasts and torso; cervical nodes drain inside the mouth as well as the head and neck; and groin nodes drain the lower limb and perineum. Ask whether you can examine other node groups, and enquire about systemic symptoms.

Lymphadenopathy in the context of typical surgical cases is discussed in Chapters 3, 5 and 7.

Differentiation of sebaceous cyst, lipoma and lymph node

It is an exam favourite to test that you can differentiate between a sebaceous cyst, a lipoma and a lymph node. This may not be as easy as it sounds, but some helpful hints are given in Table 2.1.

Ganglion*

A ganglion (a gelatinous fluid collection related to a tendon sheath or joint) is an exam favourite and makes a good case for 'on-the-spot' diagnosis. Ganglia are usually single lumps, 1–4 cm in size. They are either soft and fluctuant, or quite hard and tense, with a smooth, often rounded, outline. Ganglia are associated with a tendon sheath or joint, and are usually located around the wrist, on the dorsum of the hand or over the dorsum of the ankle. The overlying skin is usually mobile, and it may be possible to transilluminate a large ganglion.

Treatment used to be to strike the ganglion with a Bible (or other heavy object); alternatively the ganglion can be burst by injection of local anaesthetic and steroid. However, if it recurs or if the patient wishes to have the ganglion removed, surgical excision is now recommended. Ganglia are prone to recur if incompletely excised, so look for an adjacent scar.

KEY POINT

- Associated with tendon sheath or joint

Melanoma*

A pigmented skin lesion should be thought of as a melanoma in an exam, although it may well be simply a naevus (intradermal or, more rarely, junctional, compound or juvenile). Changes in size, shape or colour are the most frequently observed features of a pigmented lesion that turns out to be a melanoma. Itching, bleeding and a history of exposure to sunshine may also be noted.

Any of the following types of melanoma may turn up in the final exam: lentigo maligna melanoma (a large flat lesion, usually on an elderly person's face (Fig. 2.4), which may show areas of differing pigmentation also known as Hutchinson's melanotic freckle); superficial spreading melanoma (irregular border, areas of differing pigmentation); acral lentiginous melanoma (on the soles or palms); or nodular melanoma. Remember that all of these lesions may occur at any age (with the exception of lentigo maligna melanoma which occurs age ≥ 40 years) (Table 2.2).

You should examine the lesion and describe the following:

- Its size (in millimetres or centimetres)
- Its shape
- Its colour (there may be areas of differing pigmentation)
- Its contours
- Any satellite lesions within a few centimetres of the main melanoma
- Any metastatic nodules further away from the main melanoma

Do not forget to examine the regional lymph nodes.

You may be asked about the prognostic importance of the thickness of the melanoma, which can be measured by Clark grade I (intraepidermal) to IV (invading the subcutaneous tissues), or more usually according to the Breslow scale, which measures thickness in millimetres (Table 2.3).

Fig. 2.4 Malignant melanoma.

1 Lentigo malignant melanoma
② Preauricular nodes
③ Submandibular nodes
④ Submental nodes
⑤ Deep cervical chain
6 Enlarged jugulodigastric node

Table 2.2 Classification of melanomas
Lentigo maligna melanoma
Superficial spreading
Acral lentiginous (on the sole or palm)
Subungual
Nodular

Table 2.3 Breslow scale for melanoma	
Breslow thickness (mm)	**5-year survival rate (%)**
<1.5	<90
<1.5–3.5	<60
>3.5	<50

It is clear that the earlier a melanoma is detected and treated the better the prognosis. The golden rule is, therefore, if in doubt about a pigmented skin lesion biopsy it.

A patient with recurrent or metastatic melanoma may appear in surgical finals, because a melanoma can recur years after the original excision and metastasize widely. You should therefore ask to examine the regional lymph nodes and liver. The site of the primary lesion may be recognized by a simple scar or, commonly, a split-skin graft at the original excision site (also, look for the graft donor site, usually the thigh). Some patients may already have had regional lymph node dissection, causing a scar and also deformity of the underlying tissue. Very rarely the patient may have had an intraocular primary excised and hence have a glass eye but also liver metastases. Hence the often-repeated surgical adage (with limited relevance):

Beware the patient with a large liver and a glass eye.

KEY POINTS

- Changes in size, shape, colour
- Examine regional nodes

Basal cell carcinoma*

Basal cell carcinoma (or rodent ulcer) is usually found on the face, but occasionally on the dorsum of the hand, of elderly people with a history of exposure to sunlight. Typically, a rodent ulcer is up to 1 cm in size with a rolled, pearly edge and, usually, a central scab. You should examine for lymphadenopathy, but the rodent ulcer is, as its name suggests, locally invasive rather than metastasizing. Remember that these lesions occur in sun-damaged skin and therefore may be multiple.

Basal cell carcinoma can be equally successfully treated by radiotherapy or by surgical excision.

KEY POINTS

- Site
- Rolled pearly edge

Squamous cell carcinoma**

Squamous cell carcinoma (Fig. 2.5) may be of similar appearance to basal cell carcinoma in the early stages, and it also usually occurs in sun-exposed areas of skin. However, the edge of the lesion is red, raised and everted, and the lesion may be larger than a rodent ulcer (i.e. >1 cm). Regional lymph node metastasis may be clinically palpable. Squamous cell carcinoma may occur in the site of previous scarring (Marjolin's ulcer).

Treatment is by radiotherapy and/or surgical excision.

Squamous cell carcinoma needs to be differentiated from keratoacanthoma (benign, self-limiting, of infective origin) and solar (actinic) keratosis (premalignant, scaly lesion on sun-exposed skin of elderly people – treated with liquid nitrogen).

KEY POINTS

- Site
- Everted edge to ulcer
- Regional lymph nodes

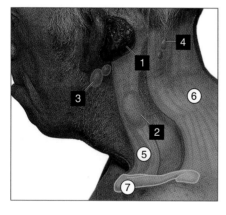

Fig. 2.5 Squamous cell carcinoma.

1 Squamous carcinoma
2 Metastatic jugulodigastric node
3 Metastatic postauricular nodes
4 Metastatic occipital nodes
⑤ Sternocleidomastoid muscle
⑥ Trapezius muscle
⑦ Clavicle

Ingrowing toenail*

An ingrowing toenail (Fig. 2.6) is a classic short case for finals. Usually the great toe is affected, often in teenagers or young men. The edges of the nail bite into the adjacent pulp tissue, causing pain, erythema and often superimposed sepsis. Sometimes the result can be an

Fig. 2.6 Ingrowing toenail.

1 Ingrowing nail
2 Inflamed skin
3 Incorrectly trimmed nail

impressive squidgy mess, but involvement may be limited to one border of one great toenail.

Treatment can be conservative, by trimming nails transversely rather than curving down into the corners of the nail bed, or by using cottonwool packs to lift up the nail. Surgical treatment can be by: simple avulsion (but the nail often ingrows again); excision of the wedge of nail and nail bed at each affected border; or removal of the nail then excision of the nail bed deep to the cuticle (Zadek's procedure). Some surgeons use phenol to cauterize the offending nail bed.

KEY POINTS

- Side of the nail grows inward as a spike
- Secondary infection in overhanging skin fold

Onychogryphosis**

In contrast to ingrowing toenails, onychogryphosis (Fig. 2.7) is usually found in elderly people and is an 'outgrowing' toenail, which may come to resemble a small horn. The lesion is said to be exacerbated by trauma or fungal infection.

It is usually treated by trimming or avulsion.

Fig. 2.7 Onychogryphosis.

Subungual melanoma***

This is an unusual form of an acral lentiginous melanoma occurring under a nail (usually the great toenail). It should form part of the differential diagnosis of any nail bed pigmentation or chronic infective process.

Dermatofibroma**

This is usually a single, pearly nodule within the skin. Dermatofibromas are about 5 mm in size, and typically occur on the lower limb, at the site of some previous, minor trauma.

Warts**

Usually occurring on the dorsum of the hand or fingers, warts (papillomas) may be an incidental finding when you examine a patient's hands. Those on the sole of the foot are known as verrucas.

Treatment involving liquid nitrogen, chemicals or surgical excision can be successful.

Fistulae**

The opening of a fistula (a communication between one epithelium-lined surface and another) may be seen as a small hole, which may weep fluid or bowel content. Fistulae may occur in the neck (branchial fistula, at the lower anterior border of the sternomastoid muscle), on the abdominal wall (from the gastrointestinal tract) or in the perianal area/perineum (particularly in Crohn's disease). It may be difficult to distinguish a fistula from a blind-ended sinus, which usually results from inadequate drainage of an abscess or indicates foreign material, such as a suture, deep inside.

Pilonidal sinus**

A pilonidal sinus is a blind-ended pit with associated hair within. The usual location is in the natal cleft in hairy young men (and occasionally in young women). It can be recognized as one or several pits, usually in the midline. There may be communications or associated scarring passing superiorly and/or laterally, adjacent to a pilonidal sinus. Rarely, a pilonidal sinus may occur in the abdominal wall or, in hairdressers, in the interdigital clefts of the hands.

Definitive treatment is by excision.

Radiotherapy changes**

Changes in the skin resulting from radiotherapy can be very subtle or quite obvious. Subtle signs are the tattoo marks (each a 1–2 mm blue/black dot) used as external markers for positioning the radiotherapy beam, which are occasionally evident on the torso or abdomen. More marked changes may be evident in the skin over the chest or head and neck, particularly if the patient was treated before the days of modern megavoltage radiotherapy. On inspection, the skin may appear pale and thickened, or quite atrophic and shiny, with telangiectasia. On palpation, the coarse or fixed skin may feel abnormal. The change from normal to treated skin may be quite abrupt at the edges of the radiation treatment fields.

Neurofibromas***

Rarely, a patient with neurofibromatosis may appear in surgical finals. The classic features are multiple neurofibromas (which may be of variable size) and café-au-lait skin lesions (milky coffee-coloured areas on the skin).

Hidradenitis suppurativa***

In this condition, the skin in the axilla, groin or perianal area appears scarred, pitted, and frequently inflamed and abscess bearing as a result of recurrent episodes of sepsis and scarring over months or years.

Treatment, if required after failed trials of antibiotics, is by excision.

Abscess/cellulitis***

You are unlikely to see an abscess in your exam, because abscesses are painful and therefore unlikely to be suitable for repeated examinations. However, the signs of inflammation (hot, tender, swollen, painful, with loss of function) would be present except in the case of a cold abscess (e.g. featuring in tuberculosis or actinomycosis). Examiners often ask you to speculate on the likely infecting organisms. The answer they expect is *Staphylococcus aureus* (in the case of a skin abscess), streptococci (in the case of cellulitis) or gut-derived organisms (in the case of abscesses in the perineal area).

Skin grafts***

Areas of skin loss that cannot be directly sutured may be closed by: a split-skin graft; a full thickness skin graft; a compound graft (such as a myocutaneous graft); or a flap. In the case of a mature split-skin graft, the underlying tissue (often muscle) is frequently almost visible through the graft, because of reduced skin thickness as a result of a lack of subcutaneous tissue. Split-skin grafts can be small postage stamp-sized pieces or extensive areas (the graft may be 'meshed' like a net to cover a large area). There should be a detectable donor site, where the donor skin has re-epithelialized, but never quite returns to a normal appearance. The donor site of a full-thickness graft may be represented simply by a linear scar or may, in turn, have been grafted with a split-skin graft. Myocutaneous flaps (latissimus dorsi, rectus abdominis, gluteal, pectoral) are unlikely to appear in finals, although they may be more likely if there is an orthopaedic trauma unit, plastic surgery unit or specialist breast unit contributing patients to finals.

Burns***

The severity of a burn depends on the injurious agent (usually heat), the duration of the injury and, for thermal burns, the temperature and speed of heat transfer (high from metal or water, lower from wood). The extent of the burns can be estimated from the size of the patient's hand (= 1% of body surface area), although this can become cumbersome – hence the 'rule of nines':

- Head and neck   9%
- Each upper limb   9% (×2)
- Each lower limb   9% × 2 (×2)
- Front of trunk   9% × 2

- Back of trunk   9% × 2
- Perineum   1%.

It is unlikely that you will be asked to examine a patient with an unhealed burn, although you may be asked about the scarring that has resulted from a full-thickness burn (with subsequent skin graft or simply healing with distorted scarring). A partial-thickness burn should heal with little residual scarring.

Others***

Spider naevae, port wine stain, pyogenic granuloma, keloid scar, hypertrophic scar, keratosis or Kaposi's sarcoma may make an appearance in surgical finals. They are generally less common as short cases than the lesions mentioned above, but merit identification in an atlas of surgical signs before you go to finals, just in case. Remember, however, that the important point is how you examine and inspect the lesion, i.e.

- Size
- Shape
- Colour
- Position
- Consistency
- Fixation
- Associated features.

KEY QUESTIONS

1. What is the difference between a sebaceous cyst and a lipoma?
2. What condition may present with lymphadenopathy?
3. Define a fistula.
4. What are the key symptoms of a melanoma?
5. What are the differences between a rodent ulcer and a squamous cell carcinoma?
6. What are the different types of skin graft?
7. How would you classify and treat burns?
8. What is a ganglion?

3

Head and neck

It is amazing how quickly you forget the anatomy that you knew so well just a few years ago! It is worth brushing up on the basic landmarks of the head and neck (Figs 3.1 and 3.2), because most head and neck cases in the exam will be swellings of some description. Stating that 'a swelling is in the submandibular triangle of the neck' will impress an examiner much more than saying 'the lump is under the chin'.

HISTORY

A general history of a patient with an abnormality of the head or neck should include the gender and age of the patient (some conditions are much more common in certain age groups), and local and systemic symptoms.

For a swelling or skin lesion, ask when it appeared, whether there has been any change in size, shape or colour, and about tenderness, redness or discharge. Has the lesion been present for a long time but changed recently? A number of developmental abnormalities may present as cystic swellings in the head and neck, usually in the second or third decades of life, e.g. a branchial cyst presents only after it has become infected or accumulated sufficient fluid to be obvious to the patient.

Systemic symptoms include: sweating/fevers (e.g. in thyroid disease, tuberculosis, lymphoma, viraemia or bacteraemia); other symptoms of thyrotoxicosis (including tremor, tachycardia, agitation, weight loss); and pain in lymphomatous nodes on alcohol ingestion. These and many other features are outlined in greater detail in the appropriate sections below.

Past medical history

Smoking, alcohol intake and exposure to radiation (particularly sunlight, radiotherapy treatment) are associated with carcinomas of the head and neck.

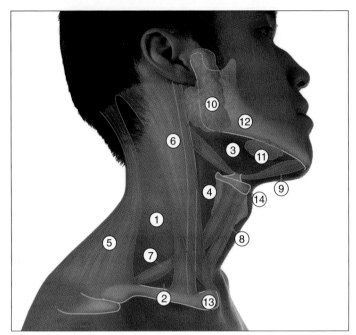

Fig. 3.1 Bony and muscular anatomy of the neck.

① Occipital triangle
② Suprascapular triangle
③ Digastric triangle
④ Carotid triangle
⑤ Trapezius muscle
⑥ Sternocleidomastoid muscle
⑦ Omohyoid muscle
⑧ Sternohyoid muscle
⑨ Digastric muscle
⑩ Parotid gland
⑪ Submandibular gland
⑫ Mandible
⑬ Clavicle
⑭ Hyoid bone

Medications may indicate the diagnosis, e.g. thyroxine for hypothyroidism, or any concomitant disease.

Family and social history

Family history may include a history of thyroid disease or malignancy (if so, where?).

Social history should include travel, contact with animals (domestic or farm), contact with known disease carriers, racial origin and home circumstances.

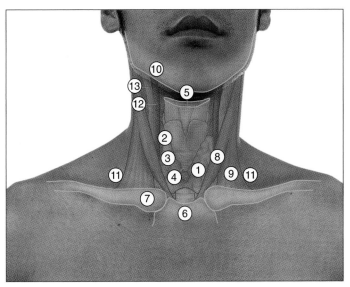

Fig. 3.2 Anterior aspect of the neck: bones, muscles, larynx and thyroid gland.

① Thyroid gland   ⑧ Sternocleidomastoid muscle – sternal head
② Thyroid cartilage   ⑨ Sternocleidomastoid muscle – clavicular head
③ Cricoid cartilage   ⑩ Mandible
④ First tracheal ring   ⑪ Supraclavicular fossae
⑤ Hyoid bone   ⑫ Carotid artery
⑥ Sternum   ⑬ Internal jugular vein
⑦ Clavicle

EXAMINATION

Exposure/position

Make sure that you have complete exposure of the head and neck down to the clavicles, and that hair does not obscure any part of the head and neck that you wish to examine. The patient will usually be sitting in a chair. A glass of water may be strategically positioned, to remind you that observing the patient swallowing can be a useful adjunct to inspection and palpation.

Inspection

Inspection is the key to identifying abnormalities in the head and neck. From a general look at the patient, gauge whether he or she shows signs of hyperthyroidism (sweating, agitation, tremor, exophthalmos) or hypothyroidism (sluggish, coarse skin, thinned hair). Are the accessory muscles of respiration being used? Looking front on at the patient, inspect from the top of the head, down the face and on to the neck and sternum: are there any visible abnormalities or scars? Then inspect each side of the head and neck in turn. Don't forget to look at the back of the neck, asking the patient to lift up the hair if necessary. Remember that lesions may lie behind the ears, or be hidden in the buccal cavity or by the tongue (Fig. 3.3), so if you do not look specifically you may miss something important.

After your initial inspection, you may want to watch what happens in certain circumstances. If you suspect a midline neck swelling or thyroid swelling, ask the patient to swallow (using the glass of water if supplied). Is there any reason to suspect facial nerve palsy (e.g. a parotid tumour or scar over the course of the facial nerve)? If so, ask the patient to show you his or her teeth, to try to whistle and to screw up the eyes (though not all three at once!), and look for weakness of one side or facial asymmetry. You may want to inspect eye movements in a patient with facial trauma (cranial nerves III and VI and the muscles they supply are particularly vulnerable to injury), or lid retraction/lid lag in someone with thyroid disease.

Point out (diplomatically, as the patient may be listening) to the examiner any skin lesions, scars, obvious lumps or swellings. Describe the:

- size
- shape
- colour
- position

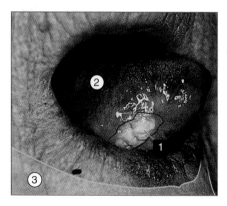

Fig. 3.3 Squamous carcinoma of the tongue.

1 Squamous cancer
② Tongue
③ Mandible

- consistency (palpation necessary)
- fixation to skin and/or deeper structures (palpation necessary)
- associated features (e.g. movement with swallowing).

Palpation

Palpation should focus on the abnormalities that you have spotted by a thorough inspection; aim to define the position of a lesion and elicit features such as fluctuance, which may help you come to a diagnosis. You may detect additional abnormalities (such as lymph nodes), which were not apparent on inspection.

The trachea (to test for tracheal deviation), occipital lymph nodes and sometimes midline neck lesions may be most readily palpated when standing in front of the patient. Similarly, buccal examination (wearing gloves) should be carried out when standing in front of the patient. The thyroid, parotid, anterior triangle, posterior triangle and supraclavicular structures are best palpated when standing behind the patient, who should be seated.

Specific points to consider on palpation include:

- Is the lump in the skin, subcutaneous tissues or muscle, or is it mobile in the neck?
- Does the lump move on swallowing?
- Is the lump pulsatile, expansile or fluctuant? (Use three fingers – two to fix the lesion in place and the third to press gently between them to test for fluctuance.)
- Can the lump be transilluminated (with a pen torch applied to the overlying skin)? This is easier to see in a darkened room, but, as an alternative, look down a tube of paper applied at one end to the skin over the illuminated lump.

Do not palpate the carotid arteries simultaneously or press too hard, in case you elicit a vagal reflex.

Percussion

Percussion in the neck may be limited to percussion over the thyroid and manubrium sternum in patients with suspected retrosternal thyroid.

Auscultation

The important structures to auscultate in the neck are the carotid vessels and the thyroid gland. A bruit in the carotid artery may be most readily heard when the patient holds his or her breath: remember to listen to both sides. A completely occluded vessel will have no flow and hence no bruit, so beware. An aortic valve murmur may be transmitted into the neck. It is said to be possible to hear a bruit over a large, hypervascular goitre – although in the exam setting this is a rare sign, listen just in case.

INVESTIGATION

Depending on the history and examination and differential diagnosis, selected investigation is required:

- Full blood count (FBV) for anaemia, elevated white cell count
- Monospot test (for Epstein–Barr virus infection)
- Plasma viscosity or erythrocyte sedimentation rate (ESR)
- Blood biochemistry, liver function tests (LFTs), proteins
- Thyroid-stimulating hormone or TSH for thyroid status (with free triiodothyronine [T_3] and thyroxine [T_4] if abnormal)
- Ultrasonography for lumps in the head and neck to determine whether they are solid or cystic and which structures they relate to
- Fine-needle aspiration (FNA) using a 19-gauge needle to aspirate a cystic lump or to aspirate a solid lump for diagnostic cytopathological examination
- Core/incisional/excisional biopsy to establish a tissue diagnosis.

TYPICAL CASES

Many of the patients you are likely to encounter in surgical finals for examination of the neck will have swellings. Remember that in the case of any lump in the neck (or elsewhere) encountered in the exam (and afterwards!) you should comment on the following:

- Size
- Shape
- Colour
- Position
- Fixation
- Consistency
- Associated features.

After inspection and palpation you should have a good idea as to what the swelling may be (Fig. 3.4). The types of commonly encountered swellings are summarized in Table 3.1.

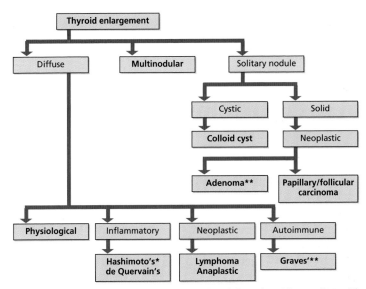

Fig. 3.4 Thyroid swellings (* may be associated with hypothyroidism and ** with hyperthyroidism).

Table 3.1 Differential diagnosis of head and neck lesions			
Congenital	Branchial cyst/branchial fistula (see Fig. 3.12) Thyroglossal cyst (see Fig. 3.13) Cystic hygroma (see Fig. 3.14) Dermoid cyst Cervical rib		
Acquired	Reticuloendothelial	Lymph node enlargement	Local Regional (see Fig. 3.9) Generalized
	Gastrointestinal	Salivary gland enlargement	Parotid (see Fig. 3.10) Submandibular (see Fig. 3.11)
	Endocrine	Thyroid	Diffuse goitre (Fig. 3.7) Solitary nodule Multinodular goitre (Fig. 3.6)
	Skin	Basal cell carcinoma Squamous cell carcinoma (see Fig. 3.15) Melanoma (see Fig. 3.16) Sebaceous cyst (see Fig. 2.2) Lipoma (see Fig. 2.3)	

ACQUIRED SWELLINGS

Thyroid enlargement*

HISTORY

Thyroid swellings (Figs 3.5–3.7) may be associated with hyperthyroidism (e.g. in Graves' disease, toxic multinodular goitre – Fig. 3.6), hypothyroidism (Fig. 3.7) (e.g. with Hashimoto's thyroiditis, iodine deficiency, drugs including lithium) or the euthyroid state (e.g. with physiological goitre, multinodular goitre, solitary nodules). It is important to ask for clues about the state of the patient's thyroid, such as sweating, agitation, tremor, tachycardia, atrial fibrillation, irritability or heat intolerance (which occur with hyperthyroidism), and pretibial myxoedema, increasing lethargy, cold intolerance, weight gain, voice changes and menstrual disturbance (which occur with hypothyroidism). Table 3.2 summarises the differences between hyperthyroidism and hypothyroidism.

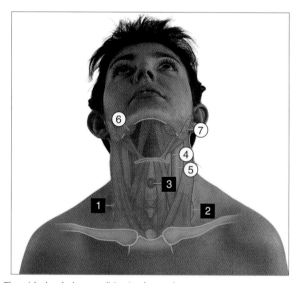

Fig. 3.5 Thyroid gland abnormalities in the neck.

1 Multinodular thyroid goitre
2 Diffuse goitre
3 Thyroglossal cyst
4 Carotid artery
5 Internal jugular vein
6 Submandibular gland
7 Parotid gland

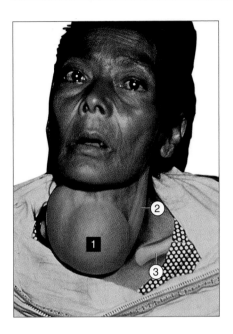

Fig. 3.6 Multinodular goitre with dominant nodule.

1 Goitre with dominant nodule
② Sternocleidomastoid muscle
③ Clavicle

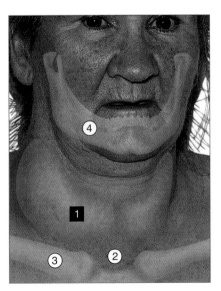

Fig. 3.7 Woman with diffuse goitre.

1 Diffuse goitre
② Sternal notch
③ Clavicle
④ Mandible

Table 3.2 Symptoms of hypothyroidism and hyperthyroidism

	Hyperthyroidism	Hypothyroidism
Demeanour	Agitated	Lethargic
Skin	Warm and sweating	Cool/dry/coarse hands
Voice	Normal	Hoarse
Pulse	Rapid ± atrial fibrillation	Slow
Weight	Reduced	Increased
Menstruation	Disrupted	Disrupted

In addition to being noted as a swelling, a large (and/or retrosternal) goitre can cause tracheal compression (with stridor), dysphonia and even dysphagia. An anaplastic carcinoma of the thyroid may cause a recurrent laryngeal nerve palsy, resulting in a hoarse voice and bovine cough. Goitres are usually painless, but pain does occur with subacute thyroiditis (de Quervain's thyroiditis), haemorrhage into a cyst, rapidly enlarging anaplastic carcinomas and, occasionally, Hashimoto's thyroiditis.

EXAMINATION

Examination of the thyroid follows the familiar scheme of inspection, palpation, percussion and auscultation, following which you will have some idea as to the likely diagnosis (see Fig. 3.4).

INSPECTION

Look for eye and skin signs of thyroid disease:

- For hyperthyroidism (Fig. 3.6): proptosis, lid retraction, lid lag, corneal oedema (chemosis), warm periphery, sweating skin, fine hand tremor and more rarely, ophthalmoplegia
- For hypothyroidism (Fig. 3.7): coarse features, periorbital puffiness, dry skin and thinned hair.

During the examination, bear in mind the possible diagnoses associated with each of multinodular goitre, diffuse enlargement and solitary nodules. Apparently diffuse enlargement suggests Graves' disease, anaplastic carcinoma, simple (deficiency) goitre, sarcoidosis or (if tender) thyroiditis. A single nodule suggests a simple cyst, a benign adenoma, or follicular or papillary carcinoma.

With the patient's neck and shoulders adequately exposed, inspect from the front and sides. Is there a single lump or is there a diffuse swelling? Decide on the position of the lump, and look for movement with swallowing – a thyroid lump moves up, then down, as the patient swallows, as a result of the envelopment of the thyroid gland in the pretracheal fascia. Consider the features applicable to any lump. The shape of a thyroid swelling will be that of a diffuse enlargement, a unilobular enlargement or a single nodule, and its size (in centimetres) should be measured. Remember to inspect (and palpate) for associated cervical lymph nodes or the attachment of the goitre to local structures. If given the opportunity, look for lid lag, ophthalmoplegia and altered reflexes. Features associated with an enlarged thyroid may include regional lymph node enlargement or a bruit.

Stand behind the patient to palpate the thyroid, and ask the patient to swallow: this is when a glass of water may be useful (try to swallow several times when you are dry mouthed and nervous). The gland's consistency is important – hard, woody glands are associated with either malignancy or thyroiditis, and fixation to the trachea indicates malignancy. Palpate for regional lymphadenopathy.

- Percuss (over the sternum for a retrosternal goitre): limb reflexes may be enhanced in hyperthyroidism or few in hypothyroidism.
- Auscultate (with the patient holding his or her breath) for the bruit of a hyperdynamic thyroid blood flow, occasionally found in Graves' disease.

INVESTIGATION

Blood tests

- Thyroid-stimulating hormone (TSH): to distinguish between biochemically hyperthyroid patients (low TSH) and thyroid failure (high TSH); this can be supplemented with triiodothyronine (T_3)/thyroxine (T_4)
- Circulating antibodies: for Hashimoto's or Graves' disease
- Calcitonin: for medullary thyroid cancer (also used to detect early cases of multiple endocrine neoplasia).

Radiology

- Chest radiograph: for a soft tissue mass in the upper mediastinum
- Thoracic outlet views: for a suspected retrosternal thyroid

- Ultrasonography: can determine whether a palpable thyroid lump is cystic or solid, and whether it is solitary or multiple
- Radionuclide scanning: can identify whether thyroid lesions are 'hot' (benign) or 'cold' (potentially malignant). Confusingly, thyroid metastases may also show up as hot nodules on scanning, because the uptake of isotope by the metastasis is greater than that by the surrounding normal tissue.

Other investigations

A fine needle can be used to obtain cells from cystic or solid lesions by aspiration for cytology.

Ultrasound visualisation of a thyroid swelling, combined with FNA cytology (FNAC), has become the investigation of choice in expert centres.

TREATMENT

The treatment of thyroid disease may be conservative (for benign, minimally enlarged, euthyroid goitre), medical (oral T_4 to correct hypothyroidism), radiotherapy (radioiodine for hyperthyroidism) or surgery (thyroid lobectomy, subtotal thyroidectomy or total thyroidectomy, depending on the condition being treated).

The complications of surgery (although rare) include recurrent laryngeal nerve palsy, superior laryngeal nerve palsy, hypocalcaemia (transient, but may be severe), tracheal compression caused by a haematoma or a thyroid storm.

SUMMARY

If you encounter a thyroid swelling in your exam, your history should include:

- Age and sex of patient
- Length of time swelling has been present/changes
- Symptoms of hypo-/hyperthyroidism
- Drugs and medicines including previous radioiodine.

Specific examination should include:

- Extent of swelling, i.e. diffuse/multinodular or uninodular
- Is there retrosternal extension?
- Is there fixation to skin or underlying structures?
- What is the consistency of the swelling?

- Are there any associated features of nerve injury/cervical lymph nodes?

General examination

- Is the patient euthyroid/hypothyroidal or hyperthyroidal?

KEY POINTS

- Clinical symptoms
- Nature of thyroid swelling (Fig. 3.4)
- TSH for thyroid status
- Ultrasonography + FNA for diagnosis of thyroid swelling.

Cervical nodes*

HISTORY

Ask about the position (Fig. 3.8) and duration of the swelling(s), and any related pain. Enquire about systemic symptoms, e.g. anorexia, malaise, sweating (sometimes at night), pain in the nodes on alcohol ingestion (in the case of lymphoma), and whether there is enlargement of other lymph node groups. Has there been any intraoral disease process such as tooth decay, or discharge from the lump(s) into the mouth or to the skin? Ask whether there have been any serious medical illnesses or surgical operations elsewhere in the past (thinking particularly of metastatic breast, lung or gastrointestinal cancer). Ask whether there has been any contact with animals or any foreign travel. Bear in mind the age and racial origin of the patient, which may point you towards the more likely diagnoses: infectious causes are more common in young people; malignancy is more likely in older people.

KEY POINT

- Symptoms and number and distribution of nodes suggest the most useful investigation(s) and likely diagnosis

---

EXAMINATION

Expose the patient's head and neck, and position him or her so as to be comfortable (usually seated) and so that you can examine him or her with ease.

Note whether there are any general features of disease (such as jaundice, cachexia), or heavily nicotine-stained fingers. Remember that

Fig. 3.8 Distribution of lymph nodes in the neck.

① Postauricular
② Preauricular
③ Occipital
④ Deep cervical chain
⑤ Jugulodigastric node
⑥ Submandibular
⑦ Submental
⑧ Superficial cervical chain
⑨ Supraclavicular
⑩ Superficial cervical chain around anterior jugular veins

⑪ Mastoid bone
⑫ Internal jugular vein
⑬ External jugular vein
⑭ Clavicle
⑮ Mandible
⑯ Trapezius
⑰ Sternocleidomastoid muscle
⑱ Parotid gland
⑲ Submandibular gland

inspection (Fig. 3.9), then palpation, should enable you to comment on the following: position and size of enlarged lymph nodes; their shape; whether they are single, multiple or matted to each other; any fixation of the glands to the overlying skin, adjacent structures, underlying muscle or each other; their consistency (soft/rubbery/hard); the colour of the overlying skin; and whether there are associated lesions such as

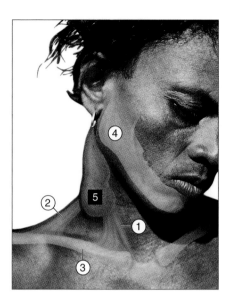

Fig. 3.9 Swollen jugulodigastric nodes.

① Sternocleidomastoid muscle
② Trapezius muscle
③ Clavicle
④ Mandible
5 Jugulodigastric nodes

generalized lymphadenopathy or intraoral lesions. Inspection of the neck should guide you to the principal node groups involved (Fig. 3.8) and to any skin tethering (e.g. at the site of a tuberculous node sinus). Always remember to inspect areas from which a lymph node may be draining – look in the mouth to see if the submental lymph node that you have just identified is caused by intraoral sepsis or intraoral carcinoma.

Palpation should be performed systematically. Stand behind the seated patient and use the pulps of your fingers gently to palpate the left and right sides simultaneously (so that you can compare them as you go along), starting anteriorly at the chin and passing posteriorly beneath the mandible. Patients often try to help you by lifting their chin but, as this has the opposite effect, you may need to remind them to drop the chin. With gentle rotating movements of your finger pulps, you should palpate even quite small nodes. At the angle of the mandible, pass inferiorly down the anterior border of sternomastoid, palpating the anterior triangle nodes. Return to the angle of the mandible and palpate the preauricular (parotid) and retroauricular regions. Move your hands inferiorly to examine the posterior triangle, and further inferiorly down to the supraclavicular fossa and then the infraclavicular fossa, before finally checking the occipital nodes. Much is made in exams of Troisier's sign, a palpable lymph node in the left supraclavicular fossa (Virchow's node). It is unusual to find this node in isolation.

INVESTIGATION

Blood tests

A FBC and ESR should be obtained. In certain circumstances it may be appropriate to check the serum for viral titres (e.g. Epstein–Barr antibodies, or HIV status after counselling) and other organisms.

Radiology

A chest radiograph may confirm the clinical diagnosis, e.g. by revealing hilar nodes, the Ghon focus of TB, bronchogenic carcinoma or secondary malignancy. Ultrasonography may differentiate nodes from other neck lumps.

Other investigations

A full examination of the nasopharynx, including laryngoscopy and possibly endoscopic examination of the upper gastrointestinal tract, should also be considered. FNA cytology and/or biopsy may provide a definitive answer as to what pathological process underlies the lymphadenopathy.

Salivary glands**

There are three major pairs of salivary glands (parotid, submandibular and sublingual), and numerous unnamed glands throughout the oral mucosa. Tumours and stones generally affect a single major gland, but viral illness and autoimmune disease may affect several or all of the glands. The features of the most commonly encountered salivary gland swellings are listed in Table 3.3.

KEY POINTS

- The history often suggests the likely diagnosis
- Tumours usually involve the parotid gland
- Calculi usually occur in the submandibular gland
- Ultrasonography (±FNA) can secure the diagnosis

HISTORY

The duration of the swelling, whether it is unilateral or bilateral and whether it increases with salivary stimulation, can all hint at the patho-

Table 3.3 Salivary gland swellings

Type of lesion	Features
Neoplastic	
Pleomorphic adenomas	Most commonly in parotid Benign/slow growth, but local recurrence if enucleated Patients usually <50 years of age
Adenolymphoma	Often soft/partially cystic Benign/slow growing Patients usually >50 years of age
Anaplastic carcinoma	Fast growing Hard and woody Invades locally Cranial nerve VII palsy Regional lymphadenopathy Retrotonsillar enlargement
Salivary calculi	Submandibular gland most commonly involved Intermittent swelling Pain
Inflammatory	
Viral (mumps)	Usually bilateral, but occasionally unilateral Painful Prodromal illness
Autoimmune	Associated with dry mouth/eyes Frequently bilateral Associated with connective tissue disease, e.g. Sjögren syndrome, Mikulicz syndrome
Acute parotitis	Associated with poor oral hygiene
Sialectasis	
Sarcoidosis	

logical process involved. The last symptom, which suggests a stone in the duct, may be associated with a gush of metallic-tasting salivary fluid as the stone falls back. Pain usually suggests an inflammatory process – the parotid in particular is invested in a dense cervical fascia, and acute enlargement can be extremely painful. Ask about systemic symptoms, such as prodromal illness, and symptoms suggestive of connective tissue disease such as joint or muscle pains, dry eyes or dry mouth.

EXAMINATION

With the patient suitably positioned and adequately exposed, visual inspection may well hint at the diagnosis, or at least suggest which gland is involved. The parotid gland is bilateral (so remember to compare the two sides), and comprises two parts: the preauricular (superficial) and retromandibular (deep to the angle of the jaw) (Fig. 3.10). The former is readily palpable, particularly when enlarged by tumour, an obstructing stone or an inflammatory process (e.g. infection by mumps virus, which may cause unilateral or bilateral swelling). Of tumours, 80% occur in the parotid and 15% in the submandibular gland, whereas 80% of obstructing stones occur in the submandibular gland and 20% in the parotid. The deep part of the parotid gland may be difficult to distinguish from the submandibular gland or from cervical lymph nodes on clinical examination, but can be affected by the same disease processes as can affect the superficial parotid.

Occasionally a parotid tumour will enlarge into the retrotonsillar space, so remember to examine inside the mouth. While looking in the mouth, visualize and then, using a gloved hand, palpate the parotid duct orifice (in the cheek opposite the upper second molar) and the submandibular duct opening (on the floor of the mouth adjacent to the frenulum of the tongue) – you may see a stone. Test the cranial nerve VII for facial nerve palsy. The facial nerve runs through the parotid gland (Fig. 3.10) and is in danger of transection during surgical explora-

Fig. 3.10 Parotid gland tumour.

1 Superficial parotid
2 Deep parotid
③ Mandible
④ Sternocleidomastoid muscle
⑤ Facial nerve

tion. Parotid tumours may also cause a nerve VII paralysis. The cervical branch of the facial nerve is closely applied to the submandibular gland, and may be damaged in surgical excision of this gland.

Palpate the parotid and submandibular glands. An abnormal submandibular gland (Fig. 3.11) is usually unilateral and should be readily palpable if the patient relaxes the chin inferiorly. Don't forget that intraoral examination (wearing gloves) to palpate the submandibular ducts and glands, and the parotid duct, is an important part of the examination of the salivary glands: say so to your examiner. After palpation of the glands, feel for regional nodal enlargement.

INVESTIGATIONS

Blood tests

Blood tests should be carried out in addition to basic haematology, biochemical and immunological studies (for viral infection or manifestations of immunological systemic disease such as rheumatoid arthritis).

Radiology

Ultrasonography may be helpful to differentiate between salivary glands and other structures in the neck. If stones in the submandibular glands are suspected, plain radiology of the floor of the mouth may be supple-

Fig. 3.11 Swollen submandibular gland.

1 Submandibular gland
2 Thyroid cartilage
3 Mandible
4 Sternocleidomastoid muscle
5 Marginal mandubular branch of facial nerve
6 External jugular vein

mented by sialograms (for which radio-opaque dye is injected via a cannula into the salivary duct to demonstrate ectatic ducts and/or obstruction).

Other investigations

FNAC or core biopsy (under local anaesthetic) has its advocates and may confirm the diagnosis, but runs the risk of a painful haematoma and implanting tumour cells.

Carotid body tumour***

This is a firm lump (which, together with the macroscopic appearance on sectioning, gives the alternative name 'potato tumour') in the course of the carotid artery. Such tumours may be bilateral and can be associated with blackouts or transient ischaemic episodes.

CONGENITAL SWELLINGS

Branchial cyst**

A branchial cyst develops because of a failure of fusion of the embryonic second and third branchial arches. It is unusual for a cyst to present before adolescence, when it is seen as a smooth rubbery swelling, bulging forwards from deep to the anterior border of the middle third of sternomastoid. Occasionally there is a branchial fistula (a communication between two epithelium-lined surfaces – Fig. 3.12) running between the tonsillar fossa and the skin at the anterior border of sternomastoid, at the junction of its middle and lower third (where it can be hidden behind clothing if the neck is not adequately exposed).

Thyroglossal cyst**

This is a remnant of the thyroglossal duct, from which the thyroid gland develops. A thyroglossal cyst (Fig. 3.13) is usually a smooth, rounded swelling located in the midline between the thyroid isthmus and the hyoid bone. It is non-tender (unless infected) and is rubbery in consistency. It moves upwards then downwards when the patient swallows, because of the attachment of the pretracheal fascia.

Ultrasonography can confirm the diagnosis. Excision may necessitate removal of the whole thyroglossal duct, which originates at the foramen caecum (at the junction of the anterior two-thirds and posterior third

Fig. 3.12 Branchial fistula.

① Sternocleidomastoid muscle
② Sternal notch
③ Mandible
④ Thyroid cartilage
⑤ Clavicle
⑥ Trachea
7 Site of fistula opening
8 Fistula tract

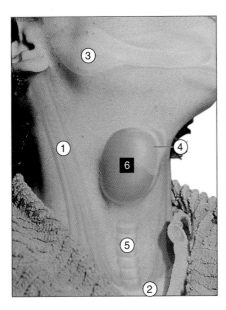

Fig. 3.13 Thyroglossal cyst.

① Sternocleidomastoid muscle
② Sternal notch
③ Mandible
④ Thyroid cartilage
⑤ Trachea
6 Thyroglossal cyst

of the tongue) and takes a convoluted course around the hyoid bone down to the isthmus of the thyroid.

Dermoid cyst***

Dermoid cysts on the head or neck are usually inclusion cysts, resulting from the sequestration of dermal cells at the site of fusion of embryonic clefts and sinuses. They present as smooth, mobile, cutaneous swellings, in the region of the supraorbital ridge (external angular dermoid cyst) or in the midline at the base of the nose or inferior to the chin (submental dermoid cyst). An implantation dermoid cyst is caused by the traumatic implantation of skin, and usually occurs elsewhere, such as on the hands or feet.

Cervical rib***

A cervical rib may be visible as a lump superior to the clavicle, with a palpable subclavian artery; usually it is not and patients present with symptoms. Most commonly these are neurological T1 and C8 dermatome pain and weakness. Vascular symptoms may result from pressure by the cervical ribs on the subclavian artery (claudication, rest pain or Raynaud's phenomenon ± signs of embolism) or the subclavian vein (swelling). Symptoms may be aggravated by bracing the shoulders and exercising the hands.

Cystic hygroma***

A cystic hygroma (Fig. 3.14) is a collection of dilated lymphatic channels, found at the base of the posterior triangle (related to the thoracic duct, if on the left side of the neck). A cystic hygroma usually presents in children as a soft, fluctuant, compressible lump, which may be large enough to occupy the base of the posterior triangle. This position is characteristic and the diagnosis is usually clinched by transillumination. A cystic hygroma is said to be 'brilliantly transilluminable'. Treatment has traditionally been excision, but recently injection of sclerosants has been successfully utilised.

Skin lesions on the head and neck*

HISTORY

It is important to ask about both the patient's age and the history of a lump. Patients with sebaceous cysts or Peutz–Jeghers syndrome may be

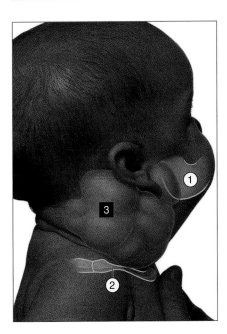

Fig. 3.14 Cystic hygroma in a baby.

① Mandible
② Clavicle
3 Cystic hygroma

young; patients with skin malignancy are often, but not exclusively, elderly. Changes in the size, shape and colour of a lesion (particularly if a melanoma is suspected), and episodes of swelling, pain and discharge, should all be explored with the patient. Prolonged exposure to sunlight (what is/was the patient's occupation?) may be aetiological in skin malignancy of the head or neck.

EXAMINATION

Once again, follow the exposure, inspection, palpation (percussion, auscultation) scheme.

Skin lesions occur on the head and neck, just as elsewhere on the body, and can be within the skin (e.g. sebaceous cyst, basal cell carcinoma, squamous cell carcinoma – Fig. 3.15 – melanoma – Fig. 3.16) or in the subcutaneous tissues (e.g. lipoma, neuroma, fibroma). Typical skin lesions of the head and neck (covered in more detail in Chapter 2) include the following:

- Sebaceous cyst★ (in the skin has a punctum)
- Lipoma★ (subcutaneous, appears fluctuant)
- Melanoma★ (change in size, shape or colour)

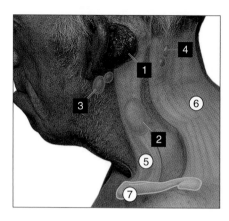

Fig. 3.15 Squamous cell carcinoma.

1 Squamous carcinoma
2 Metastatic jugulodigastric node
3 Metastatic postauricular nodes
4 Metastatic occipital nodes
⑤ Sternocleidomastoid muscle
⑥ Trapezius muscle
⑦ Clavicle

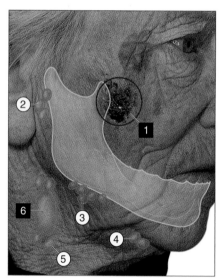

Fig. 3.16 Malignant melanoma.

1 Lentigo malignant melanoma
② Preauricular nodes
③ Submandibular nodes
④ Submental nodes
⑤ Deep cervical chain
6 Enlarged jugulodigastric node

- Basal cell carcinoma★ (a rolled pearly edge, typically develops over the midface); may also be associated with other hyperkeratotic lesions and solar keratosis
- Squamous cell carcinoma★★ (remember neck nodes).

In addition, beware of scarring from burns, surgery or radiotherapy (often with telangiectasias in skin that is thin and shiny (Fig. 3.10) or coarse and thickened). Remember that squamous carcinoma can arise in scar tissue (when it is called Marjolin's ulcer).

Despite their rarity in the real world, the perioral freckles of Peutz–Jeghers syndrome (which also includes multiple benign polyps in the small bowel) and telangiectasia around the mouth, lips and gums in hereditary haemorrhagic telangiectasia (associated also with gastrointestinal bleeding) are such classic symptoms that they can be used for spot diagnoses.

A range of 'medical' conditions may also manifest themselves on the skin of the head and neck, including jaundice, anaemia, psoriasis, malar flush of mitral valve disease, herpes zoster and xanthelasma.

Carcinomas of the oral cavity***

Squamous carcinoma of the lip often presents as a non-healing sore and should be a differential diagnosis of any chronic wound on the lips. The classic appearance is a rolled ulcer, usually in a smoker (often a pipe smoker).

Cancers of the floor of the mouth or tongue (Fig. 3.3) are also associated with smoking and may be ulcerated and associated with leukoplakia. Remember to palpate bimanually if not too tender and to check for fixation of the tongue. Cervical nodes are frequently enlarged.

Eye signs*

In surgical finals, eye signs of disease elsewhere are usually caused by a nerve palsy (usually nerve III, rarely nerve VI, and occasionally Horner syndrome) or are related to thyroid disease (e.g. lid lag, exophthalmos, ophthalmoplegia).

HISTORY

Symptoms of hyperthyroidism (Fig. 3.17), head or facial trauma, or smoking (e.g. Pancoast syndrome) may give a hint as to the condition responsible for the eye signs. Pancoast syndrome is the spectrum of symptoms and signs caused by a bronchogenic carcinoma at the apex of the lung (sometimes called Pancoast's [bronchogenic] carcinoma), including severe pain (which may radiate down the arm), Horner syndrome and rib erosion.

EXAMINATION

Initial inspection may enable you to spot the diagnosis in some cases, e.g. the proptosis of thyrotoxicosis, ipsilateral miosis and ptosis

Fig. 3.17 Appearance of the eyes in hyperthyroidism – proptosis, lid retraction, chemosis.

in Horner syndrome (enophthalmos and the ipsilateral loss of sweating of the face may be less obvious), nerve III palsy (ipsilateral large pupil, ptosis, downward and outward gaze) and subconjunctival haemorrhage. Less immediately apparent features (but common and still worthy of mention to your examiner) include arcus senilis and xanthelasmas.

Beware of the glass eye: you would not be the first exam candidate to be caught out. A glass eye may be a very good colour match to the normal eye, but does not have the full range of movement. Also, there will be no pupillary reflex to light or accommodation!

Visual field assessment, fundoscopy and detailed examination of the cranial nerves are usually reserved for the medical part of final exams, or postgraduate exams.

INVESTIGATION

It may be appropriate to mention laboratory tests for thyroid disease, lipid/cholesterol levels, diabetes or other metabolic disorders, depending on your clinical findings.

A chest radiograph may detect a lesion causing Horner syndrome (e.g. ipsilateral Horner syndrome caused by invasion of the cervical sympathetic plexus as a result of carcinoma of the bronchus).

Facial nerve palsy***

Facial (nerve VII) nerve palsy can be caused by either a lower motor neuron lesion (typically secondary to trauma, surgery to the parotid, tumour of the parotid or Bell's palsy) or an upper motor neuron lesion (in which case the frontalis muscle is spared as a result of bilateral cortical representation). A lower motor neuron lesion may affect only the branches transected (test the orbicularis oris, orbicularis oculi and frontalis muscles).

Cushingoid facies*

A cushingoid facies in surgical finals is usually iatrogenic. Patients receiving steroids for chronic inflammatory disease (e.g. arthritis, inflammatory bowel disease), immunosuppression or autoimmune disease may develop cushingoid features – they are rarely the result of endogenous excess steroid production.

Signs of this condition include a moon face with red rounded cheeks, facial hirsutism, easily bruised, fragile skin, striae (e.g. on the abdominal wall and thighs), proximal myopathy, and buffalo hump (which may be accentuated by osteoporotic collapse of the spine).

Miscellaneous

Occasionally in exams you may be asked to comment on a central line or a tracheostomy.

CENTRAL VENOUS LINES*

A central venous line is inserted either to allow monitoring of central venous pressure or to allow venous access – most commonly for parenteral nutrition or chemotherapy. The tip of the line itself should lie in the superior vena cava at the junction with the right atrium, where it should be visible on a chest radiograph. A venous line is a potential portal for infection (infection may be reduced by inserting the line through a skin tunnel), so the line should always be handled with an aseptic technique.

The complications associated with a central line relate first to its insertion and second to its management. During insertion it is possible to damage anatomically related structures in the neck, i.e. the apex of the lung/pleura, the subclavian artery, branches of the brachial plexus or even the thoracic duct (on the left side). Pneumothorax and haemothorax are worth remembering. It is also possible to cause an air embolism, or embolism of the tip of the line if it is sheared off during insertion. If the line is in so far that it lies within the atrium, it may precipitate dysrhythmias. Longer-term complications are usually related to infection of the line, but it is possible for the tip of the line to puncture vascular structures or to precipitate a subclavian thrombosis. The complications of TPN (total parenteral nutrition) therapy (electrolyte imbalance, hyperosmolarity, hyperammonaemia, metal ion deficiency) or chemotherapy may occur.

TRACHEOSTOMY***

A tracheostomy tube is inserted through the upper two tracheal cartilages, inferior to the cricoid cartilage, to allow access to the airway for ventilation, to reduce respiratory dead space and to allow bronchial suction. It is most often performed electively in patients who require prolonged ventilation, because it is easier to manage and less traumatic than an orotracheal tube, which would pass through the vocal folds. Patients who have undergone a laryngectomy will have a permanent tracheostomy. The principal complications of a tracheostomy are: bleeding or airway obstruction, particularly at the time of insertion; drying of bronchial secretions (if the inspired air is not humidified), which may lead to pulmonary collapse or blockage of the tracheostomy; damage to the tracheal wall (from the cuff on the tracheostomy tube), with late stenosis; displacement of the tube into the neck (with resultant surgical emphysema); or the tube falling out completely.

HEAD INJURY GUIDELINES

You may be asked about the advice you would give to a patient with a minor head injury. Written advice should be given to a relative or friend of any patient who has suffered even a minor head injury. The patient should not:

- be left alone
- be allowed to drive a vehicle or ride a bicycle
- drink alcohol.

After a head injury, a patient who develops any of the following symptoms must be seen by a GP or taken to a hospital as soon as possible:

- Confusion or irritability
- Drowsiness or difficult to rouse
- Severe or progressive headache

- Blurred or double vision
- Vomiting
- Dizziness
- Any form of muscle weakness
- Slurring or loss of speech
- A fit or seizure.

Clearly, if a patient has neurological symptoms or signs or a skull fracture (Fig. 3.18), further investigation by CT scan should be suggested.

Fig. 3.18 Transverse skull fracture across frontal and temporal bones.

1. What are the causes of the following types of thyroid enlargement:
   - single nodule?
   - multinodular?
   - diffuse?
2. What are the causes of enlargement of the parotid gland and of the submandibular gland?
3. What are the causes of cervical lymphadenopathy:
   - limited to the neck?
   - as part of a systemic lymphadenopathy?
4. What congenital swellings can occur and where are they sited in the head and neck?
5. What are the features of the following:
   - a sebaceous cyst?
   - a lipoma?
   - a basal cell carcinoma?
   - a squamous cell carcinoma?
   - a malignant melanoma?
6. What are the causes of a nerve VII lesion:
   - upper motor neuron?
   - lower motor neuron?
7. What are the indications for and complications of the following:
   - a tracheostomy?
   - a central venous line?
8. How would you advise a patient after a head injury?

4

Chest

In surgical exams you are less likely to be asked to examine the cardiac or respiratory systems in detail than in medical finals. However, surgically relevant features such as signs of cardiac, pulmonary or gastro-oesophageal surgery and signs of surgically important pulmonary or pleural disease do form part of surgical finals. You should remember that significant cardiopulmonary disease may well limit the treatment options in certain patients; this may be a central point in the discussion following your long case. For example, you may be faced with a patient who gives a typical history of biliary colic but who also has severe chronic obstructive pulmonary disease; the examiner may well quiz you on the risks of surgery and on how potential problems in this patient could be averted. A history of angina, hypertension, myocardial infarction or aortic stenosis places the patient at increased risk of a further cardiac event or even death in surgical practice. Surgical intervention within 6 months of a myocardial infarction, and particularly within 6 weeks, places the patient at high risk of a further, potentially fatal, myocardial infarction.

The American Society of Anesthesiologists (ASA) has developed a grading system that indicates, on the basis of the severity of pre-existing disease (often cardiorespiratory), a patient's risk of death as a result of surgery. In simplified form:

- ASA1: normal
- ASA2: mild-to-moderate systemic disturbance
- ASA3: severe systemic disturbance
- ASA4: life-threatening systemic disorder
- ASA5: moribund patient with little chance of survival.

You may be asked to examine the chest of a patient in surgical finals: this usually means just that. There is a subtle distinction between being asked to examine the chest and being asked to examine the respiratory system or cardiovascular system (in which case you should start with the hands!), so make sure you listen to what your examiner asks.

HISTORY

The principal respiratory symptoms are cough, sputum, haemoptysis, breathlessness, chest pain and wheeze. The main cardiac symptoms are chest pain, breathlessness, ankle swelling and palpitations. These symptoms may all be significant in assessing a patient's suitability for surgery and, if any are present, determine their severity. Does the patient get breathless when running for a bus, walking briskly or walking short distances, or on minimal exertion such as dressing?

Symptoms of diseases of the respiratory system relevant to surgical practice include sharp (pleuritic) chest pain, shortness of breath and haemoptysis. These can be caused by infections (e.g. pneumonia, empyema, bronchiectasis, tuberculosis), tumours (e.g. primary lung carcinoma, secondaries), vascular problems (e.g. pulmonary infarction/embolism, heart failure) or trauma (e.g. fractured ribs). Ask about any history of thoracic surgery (e.g. lung or pleural resection, surgical pneumothorax for anti-tubercle surgery), midline sternotomy (for a coronary artery bypass graft [CABG] or other cardiac procedures) or left thoracotomy (for mitral valve replacement).

EXAMINATION

Think, as you examine the chest, what might be the underlying problem. Is there a unilateral condition (e.g. pleural effusion, lobar pneumonia)? Is there a bilateral condition (e.g. bilateral crepitations of heart failure)? Are there any clues? There may be signs of intrathoracic disease elsewhere, particularly in the hands (e.g. finger clubbing – Fig. 4.1 – palmar erythema, radial pulse); head and neck (e.g. lymph nodes, jugular venous pressure); abdomen (e.g. liver) and lower limbs (e.g. peripheral oedema).

Fig. 4.1 Finger clubbing.

Exposure/position

Expose the torso so that it can be fully examined. For a chest examination, the traditional position for the patient is sitting propped up on pillows at a 45° angle. Alternatively, you may be presented with a patient sitting in a chair. When examining the chest, compare right with left and front with back.

Inspection

Inspection of the chest should include the use of your ears for the tell-tale clicking of a prosthetic heart valve (usually mitral or aortic). Look for and comment on the presence of any deformities (e.g. kyphoscoliosis) or surgical scars. There may also be evidence of other surgical procedures, e.g. central, feeding or chemotherapy lines, chest drains or cardiac pacemaker (although all of these are sometimes inserted by physicians).

Assess the patient's respiratory rate and look for signs of laboured breathing, including the use of the accessory respiratory muscles, the intercostal muscles being drawn in and chest expansion. With the patient propped up at 45°, look for the jugular venous pulse wave and the height (pressure) of the filled vein. Look for signs of superior vena cava obstruction – swelling of the conjunctivae, face, neck and upper limbs, visible collateral veins and prominent jugular veins. Check the sputum pot for the colour of the sputum and the presence of blood.

Palpation

Palpation should begin by examining the trachea for deviation to one side (pushed by a growth or intrapleural expansion, or pulled as a result of collapse or contraction to the side of the disease process). Test for chest expansion, both anteriorly and posteriorly – poor expansion is a sign of a disease process on that side of the chest (bilateral in chronic obstructive airway disease). Feel for vocal fremitus.

Percussion

Percuss down each rib space (don't forget the apices or the midaxillary line, and remember that the liver lies on the right-hand side, up to the fourth intercostal space). Where does the percussion note change from resonant to dull?

Auscultation

After checking the tracheal position, testing for expansion and percussing the chest, you should have some idea of whether you are going to find a unilateral or bilateral abnormality when you listen to the lung fields. Feel for the apex beat, which may be displaced as a result of intrathoracic disease from its position of the fifth intercostal space in the midclavicular line.

Auscultate for breath sounds using the bell of the stethoscope, listening for crackles (fine/coarse/clear with coughing?), bronchial breathing and, where indicated, whispering pectoriloquy (ask the patient to say 1–1–1). You may hear bowel sounds when you examine the chest of a surgical patient, as a result of a hiatus hernia or after gastro-oesophageal resection and reconstruction.

INVESTIGATIONS

In addition to the basic biochemical and haematological investigations, chest radiology (posterior/anterior film and lateral view) plays a particularly important role in confirming the clinical diagnosis, but it is essential to know the normal radiological outline (Fig. 4.2).

Spirometry, to measure forced expiratory volume in 1 second (FEV_1), forced vital capacity (FVC) and the FEV_1:FVC ratio, can be useful for comparing a patient's pulmonary function with that expected for their height and gender. Arterial blood gas measurement will indicate the arterial Po_2 and Pco_2 and any acid–base imbalances.

Do not forget that sputum cytology, needle aspiration of an effusion and bronchoscopy may contribute useful information about pulmonary or pleural diseases. An ECG, echocardiography and radiological imaging (e.g. after cardiac catheterization) may be useful in the diagnosis of cardiac disease.

TYPICAL CASES

Pleural effusion*

HISTORY

The history should include details of cardiac and respiratory symptoms and treatment, and enquiries about previous medical conditions (such as rheumatic fever) and surgical operations, particularly for cancer. The

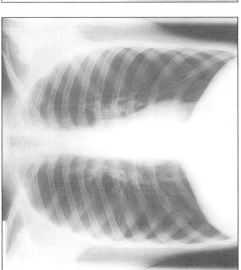

Fig. 4.2 Normal posteroanterior (PA) chest radiograph on deep inspiration.

① Trachea ③ Pulmonary vessels ⑤ Diaphragm
② Aortic arch ④ Left ventricle

lungs and pleurae are favoured sites for metastatic disease from epithelial cancers.

EXAMINATION (Table 4.1)

On inspection, the patient may look unwell (e.g. cachectic as a result of cancer). There may be signs of a previous aspiration or chest drainage procedure (e.g. bruising, a needle puncture or an Elastoplast), and chest expansion may be diminished on the affected side. Palpation may reveal reduced expansion, and on percussion there may be a stony, dull percussion note over the effusion (large unilateral effusions are easier to detect than small bilateral effusions). On auscultation, breath sounds should be absent over the effusion, although there may be bronchial breathing at the top of the effusion.

INVESTIGATIONS

A standard PA (posteroanterior – Fig. 4.3) chest radiograph, supplemented by a lateral view (Fig. 4.4), should confirm the presence of a pleural effusion by demonstrating loss of the costophrenic angle on the affected side and a homogeneous shadowing with a border that is concave upwards. Aspiration of the pleural cavity (under ultrasound

Table 4.1 Features of right pleural effusion		
	Right	**Left**
Chest expansion	Reduced	Normal
Percussion note	Stony dull over effusion	Normal
Breath sounds	Absent or decreased (occasionally bronchial)	Normal
Added sounds	None	Normal
Vocal resonance	Absent or decreased	Normal

Fig. 4.3 Pleural effusion.

① Heart   **2** Pleural effusions   ③ Diaphragm

guidance if it is a small effusion) enables cytological, biochemical and bacteriological analysis of the fluid, which may be straw coloured or blood stained. The protein content of the aspirate will indicate whether this is an exudate or a transudate.

DIAGNOSIS

If you are asked 'What are likely causes of a pleural effusion?', start with the most common and therefore the most likely diagnosis (Fig. 4.5). In surgical finals, exudates (protein > 30 g/l) are more common than transudates. Exudates may be caused by primary tumours (e.g. bronchogenic

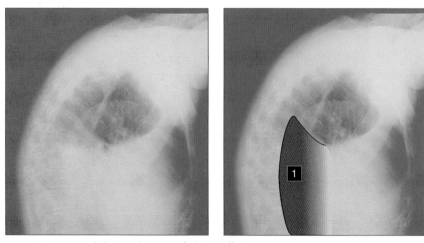

Fig. 4.4 Lateral chest radiograph of pleural effusion.

1 Pleural effusion

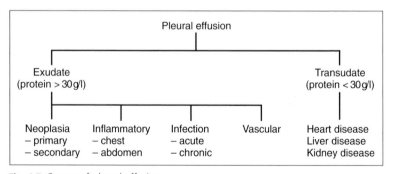

Fig. 4.5 Causes of pleural effusion.

carcinoma, mesothelioma), secondary tumours (e.g. a malignant pleural effusion resulting from breast, lung, ovarian or gastrointestinal cancer), infection within the chest (e.g. pneumonia, tuberculosis) or, rarely, by vascular lesions such as pulmonary emboli. Exudates may also be secondary to intra-abdominal inflammation or sepsis (e.g. pancreatitis, subphrenic abscess). A transudate (protein < 30 g/l) suggests a medical cause, particularly heart failure, cirrhosis or nephrotic syndrome.

Bronchogenic carcinoma**

Although lung cancers are depressingly common in clinical practice, you are far more likely to encounter one in your medical than in your surgical exams. This diagnosis should be considered for patients who are middle-aged or older and have haemoptysis or a persistent cough – particularly if they are smokers. Other clinical presentations may indicate more advanced disease, e.g. involving malignant pleural effusions or lymph node metastases. A bovine cough may be a result of compression of the left recurrent laryngeal nerve by a hilar tumour. An unusual presentation occurs when an apical tumour (which may be visible on the chest radiograph – Fig. 4.6) erodes into the first rib, causing pain and weakness in the arm in association with unilateral ptosis, miosis, enophthalmos and hypohydrosis (Horner syndrome); this combination of tumour and Horner syndrome is known as Pancoast syndrome.

Fig. 4.6 Right Pancoast's tumour.

HISTORY (Table 4.2)

If you suspect a lung tumour, ask the patient about occupation, previous lung disease and smoking.

EXAMINATION

On inspection, look for signs that may support your diagnosis: nicotine-stained fingers, finger clubbing (see Fig. 4.1), signs of cachexia and, more rarely, superior vena cava obstruction caused by mediastinal disease. Listen for evidence of recurrent laryngeal nerve paralysis. On palpation, percussion and auscultation, look for tracheal deviation and chest signs indicating a pleural effusion or pulmonary collapse. Palpate for cervical lymph nodes, rib metastases and hepatomegaly resulting from metastatic disease.

INVESTIGATIONS

As in the case of most chest problems, along with basic haematology, PA (Fig. 4.7) and lateral chest radiographs, sputum cytology and bronchoscopy (with brushings, lavage and/or biopsy) should aim to establish the diagnosis. Radiological staging may include CT or MRI.

TREATMENT

Surgical resection is rarely possible but offers the prospect of cure for early stage lesions. Combination chemotherapy or chemoradiotherapy and symptom relief are the mainstays of palliative treatment.

Pneumonia**

A patient with resolving pneumonia may be considered suitable for surgical finals. Pneumonia may be in the differential diagnosis for upper abdominal pain or may follow surgical treatment.

Table 4.2 Features of right bronchial carcinoma		
	Right	**Left**
Chest expansion	Reduced	Normal
Percussion note	Dull over affected part of lung	Normal
Breath sounds	Bronchial over affected part of lung	Normal
Added sounds	Crepitations and rhonchi over affected part of lung	Normal
Vocal resonance	May be increased over affected part of lung	Normal

Fig. 4.7 Bronchial carcinoma.

① Heart ② Bronchogenic carcinoma ③ Consolidation and lung collapse ④ Bilateral pleural effusion ⑤ Diaphragm

HISTORY

Remember to ask about the duration of cough and productivity (sputum, blood), smoking and enforced immobility resulting from other medical conditions or surgical operations; chronic pulmonary conditions predisposing to pneumonia (e.g. chronic obstructive airway disease) also provide useful clues as to the likely underlying diagnosis.

EXAMINATION (Table 4.3)

On inspection, look for central cyanosis, increased respiratory rate, perspiration, an oxygen mask or a nebulizer.

On palpation, examine for clamminess, for tracheal deviation (towards pulmonary collapse and consolidation secondary to pneumonia) and chest expansion.

On percussion, listen for dullness over the affected lower, mid or upper zone (for lobar pneumonia) or the whole lung field (for bronchopneumonia).

On auscultation, listen for bronchial breathing, crepitations (fine or more commonly coarse crackles) and wheeze (rhonchi) over the affected lung region (Figs 4.8 and 4.9).

INVESTIGATION

Investigations include full blood count (for raised white cell count), plasma viscosity/erythrocyte sedimentation rate (ESR), arterial blood gases and chest radiography (Figs 4.8 and 4.9).

TREATMENT

Humidified oxygen, nebulized bronchodilators, physiotherapy and appropriate antibiotics (administered by the oral or intravenous route) are used in treatment. Exacerbating factors such as cigarette smoking should be stopped.

Table 4.3 Features of right middle lobe pneumonia		
	Right	**Left**
Chest expansion	? reduced	Normal
Percussion note	Dull over midlobe	Normal
Breath sounds	Bronchial	Normal
Added sounds	Crepitations and rhonchi	Normal
Vocal resonance	Increased	Normal

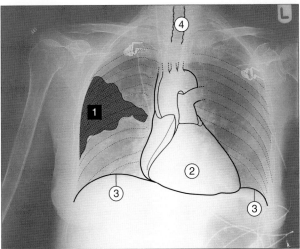

Fig. 4.8 Posteroanterior (PA) chest radiograph of pneumonia.

1 Middle lobe pneumonia   ③ Diaphragm
② Heart and great vessels   ④ Trachea

Heart valves**

Most open cardiac surgery involves Coronary Artery Bypass Graft (CABG) or valve replacement, although less invasive methods, particularly those practised by radiologists and cardiologists, have become increasingly common. Patients who have or are due to undergo heart

Fig. 4.9 Lateral radiograph of pneumonia.

1 Middle lobe pneumonia
② Right diaphragm
③ Left diaphragm
④ Heart

surgery generally fall into one of two groups: young patients who have congenital cardiac problems or have suffered infective endocarditis with valve destruction, and older patients in whom the predominant underlying pathology is degenerative vascular disease and/or a past history of rheumatic fever.

HISTORY

Ask direct questions about the patient's current and past cardiac symptoms, including breathlessness, angina, symptoms of peripheral vascular disease, and strokes(s). Ask about current and previous medications. Also ask specific questions about rheumatic fever, hypertension, myocardial infarction and investigative procedures. Most patients have had echocardiography (ultrasonography of the heart, including the valves, for structure and function) or coronary and/or cardiac angiography (performed through percutaneous puncture of the femoral artery before surgery), and may be quite knowledgeable about their investigations and the results. Patients usually also know the type of valve (mechanical or porcine graft) that has been used and may be able to state the make.

EXAMINATION

Estimate the patient's age and assess his or her general health: an obese, elderly patient is unlikely to have significant congenital heart disease, but is likely to have ischaemic heart disease, perhaps rheumatic heart disease or a pacemaker.

The upper half of the patient's body should be exposed, and traditionally the patient is examined sitting propped up at 45°. Inspection of the torso from the front and sides will reveal surgical scars such as a midline sternotomy scar (usually indicating CABG), often accompanied by scars in the epigastrium, from drainage tubes. The left thoracic approach for valve surgery and associated drain sites is usually clearly visible – if you take the trouble to inspect the left chest wall! While inspecting, listen for the rhythmic clicking of a prosthetic valve and, if you hear it, comment on it to the examiner. During inspection you may see the jugular venous pressure (JVP) (with the patient sitting propped up at 45°), and the apex beat may be visible.

Before auscultation, take the patient's hand and feel the pulse for rate, rhythm and character. Then examine for the JVP (if not already visible), systolic and diastolic blood pressures, apex beat (the fifth intercostal space in the midclavicular line) and valvular thrills.

Auscultation begins before you use the stethoscope: that irritating click (which may be regular or irregular) may turn out to be the patient's heart valve, not someone's watch! Any mechanical prosthetic valve will probably have a deafening click when you listen with a stethoscope. Remember the position of the heart and valves on the anterior chest wall, the sites for auscultation and radiation of sounds (Fig. 4.10). Use the diaphragm of the stethoscope to auscultate the heart except when seeking a mitral stenotic murmur. Cardiac murmurs are traditionally medical territory, but for a surgeon's guide to the common murmurs see Table 4.4.

(a)

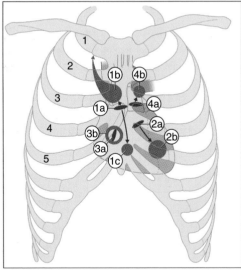

(b)

Fig. 4.10 (a) Cardiac anatomy in relation to the chest wall. (b) Position of heart valves and sites for auscultation.

1a Aortic valve

1b Aortic stenosis murmur area

1c Aortic regurgitation murmur area

2a Mitral valve

2b Mitral murmur area

3a Tricuspid valve

3b Tricuspid murmur area

4a Pulmonary valve

4b Pulmonary stenosis murmur area

5 Right atrium

6 Right ventricle

7 Left ventricle

8 Left atrial appendage

9 Aorta

10 Pulmonary artery

11 Superior vena cava

12 Fifth intercostal space (apex beat)

Table 4.4 Cardiac murmurs

Condition	Type of murmur
Aortic stenosis	Ejection systolic murmur Radiates to carotids
Aortic regurgitation	Early diastolic murmur Left sternal edge Best heard with the patient leaning forward, on expiration
Mitral stenosis	Mid-diastolic murmur At apex
Mitral regurgitation	Pansystolic murmur At apex Radiates to axilla Best heard with the patient in the left lateral position, using the bell of the stethoscope

INVESTIGATIONS

In addition to urine testing (for glucose) and basic haematology and biochemistry, the mainstays of cardiology are the ECG and, primarily, echocardiography (which can detect many abnormalities in the structure and function of the heart, including the valves).

Chest radiographs (PA and lateral) can be valuable for revealing cardiac size, shape and outline, a pacemaker, valve replacement or sternal wiring (Fig. 4.11) as well as lung field and pleural abnormalities. More advanced imaging (e.g. involving cardiac catheterization, coronary angiography, radioisotope scanning for cardiac function) may be considered if available.

Chest drains**

A patient with a chest drain may show up in finals. The first thing you have to do is to recognize he or she has a chest drain. You may think that this sounds simple, but it is surprising what people have thought chest drains are in the heat of an exam. A chest drain comes from an intercostal space and goes to a collecting bottle, with the end of the tube beneath the surface of the fluid (Fig. 4.12). When the patient coughs or breathes, the fluid within the drainage tube should move with the changing intrapleural pressure. If there is bubbling when the patient exhales, there is a persisting pneumothorax.

(a)   (b)

Fig. 4.11 Chest radiograph of pacemaker.

1 Sternotomy wires   ⑤ Trachea
2 Pacing wire   ⑥ Aorta
3 Pacemaker   ⑦ Left ventricle
4 Aortic valve replacement

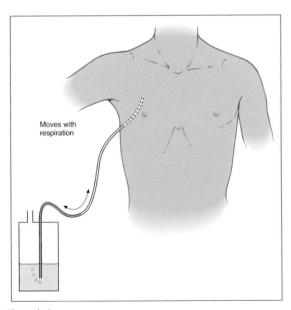

Fig. 4.12 Chest drain.

If you are confronted with a chest drain, you will almost certainly be asked 'How should this be connected up?'. The answer is that the end of the drainage tube must be under the surface of the fluid in the collecting bottle, and the bottle must be kept below the drainage site. However, one-way valve systems exist, which have the same effect. If the patient has to be moved, the tube should be double-clamped close to the patient in case it becomes detached or fluid siphons into the patient (if the bottle is placed higher than the patient).

Chest drains may be inserted to drain air (e.g. in pneumothorax), fluid (e.g. in pleural effusion), pus (e.g. in empyema) or blood (e.g. in haemothorax) (Table 4.5).

Pneumonectomy***

Pneumonectomy or pulmonary lobectomy is usually performed either for benign, inflammatory, pulmonary conditions (e.g. bronchiectasis, TB) or for malignancy (usually primary carcinoma of the lung, but sometimes isolated lung metastases).

HISTORY

Given the opportunity, the patient will often help considerably by telling you what operation has been done. The history should include particular attention to the drugs or chemotherapy the patient has had, which will often lead to the diagnosis.

Table 4.5 Positioning and use of chest drains

Condition	Position/purpose of chest drain
Pleural effusion	Usually inserted in the most gravity-dependent part of the pleural space, usually in the midaxillary line
Pneumothorax	Usually in the midclavicular line, in the second intercostal space. If there is bubbling, low pressure suction may be needed
Postoperative	Post-thoracotomy, one or two chest drains are usually inserted to prevent air or fluid collections
Empyema	Site of drain will depend on that of the collection. If pus is not draining, a rib resection may be needed
Trauma	Blood and/or air in the pleural cavity should be drained via the fifth intercostal space in the midaxillary line

EXAMINATION

Inspection will reveal the surgical scars and chest deformity that may result from surgery or the disease process. Remember to examine the trachea for deviation and to palpate the ribs for metastases. Percussion and auscultation should be used to detect the extent of the anatomical distortion after surgery.

INVESTIGATIONS

As in the case of most pulmonary problems, blood tests and radiology are useful investigations.

KEY QUESTIONS

1. What are the signs and causes of a pleural effusion?
2. What are the possible symptoms and signs of a bronchogenic carcinoma?
3. What are typical symptoms or signs of pneumonia?
4. What signs are found on inspection and auscultation of a patient with mitral valve replacement?
5. Where would you listen for aortic and mitral valve murmurs, and what would you expect to hear?

5

Breast

As breast cancer is a common condition (affecting 1 in 11 women in the UK), it appears commonly in surgical finals, in a patient with either primary cancer before surgery or (for longer cases) treated breast cancer. Patients with a fibroadenoma, cysts, nipple discharge or an abscess are also drafted into surgical finals.

HISTORY

The history should include questions related to the specific breast complaint on each side.

Lump

When was it first noted? How has it changed since then? What is its position, shape and mobility, and is it tender? Is there more than one? Is there any cyclical variation (e.g. increase in size before menses, decrease after menses)? Are there any other lumps (e.g. in the axilla)?

Skin changes

These include redness, swelling, peau d'orange (orange skin) appearance and eczema of the nipple (especially if unilateral and no eczema elsewhere, when there is a need to exclude Paget's disease, intradermal cancer, of the nipple).

Nipple retraction

If unilateral, asymmetrical and distorting, it may result from an underlying cancer.

Nipple discharge

Ask if single or multiple, what colour it is, and whether blood stained (single-duct blood-stained nipple discharge may be the result of duct papilloma or carcinoma) or galactorrhoea (milky).

Pain

Are changes cyclical or acyclical (i.e. no changes with menses)? Is pain unilateral or unifocal?

Other relevant history

- Age (Fig. 5.1)
- Menopausal status
- Menstrual history
- Parity
- Hormonal medications
- Gynaecological history
- Family history of breast cancer.

General health questions

- Past history of medical conditions
- Surgical operations

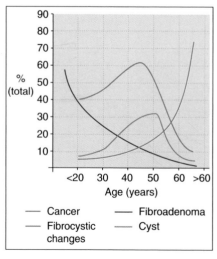

Fig. 5.1 Some types of breast lump are more common at certain ages as a percentage of all lumps at that age.

- Medications
- Allergies
- Smoking (associated with inflammatory processes in the breast)
- Symptoms suggestive of metastatic disease: breathlessness, musculoskeletal aches, tiredness, anorexia.

BREAST EXAMINATION

Exposure

With a chaperone present (particularly if you are male), ask the woman for permission to examine her and request that she removes her clothing from the upper half of her body. Wash your hands.

Inspection (Fig. 5.2)

Note that the size, shape and ptosis of the breast vary markedly between individuals and, for each woman, change with the monthly cycle, pregnancy and age.

With the woman sitting, naked to waist (Fig. 5.2a), ask her to raise her arms above her head and lean forward (Fig. 5.2b), then with her

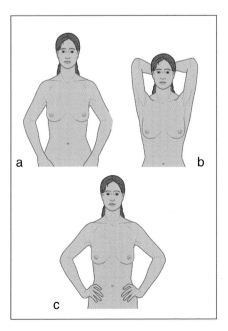

Fig. 5.2 Patient positioning for inspection of changes in breast contour.

hands on her hips to tense the pectoral muscles (Fig. 5.2c). These actions accentuate skin contour or dimpling changes (Fig. 5.3) caused by underlying breast pathology.

Look for surgical scars (which may be difficult to spot in the skin creases or around the nipple), signs of previous radiotherapy (telangiectasia, skin tattoo, thin, shiny or thickened coarse skin) or the encrusted eczematous nipple of Paget's disease.

Palpation (Fig. 5.4)

With the patient as comfortable as possible, lying flat on a couch or bed with one pillow, examine each breast systematically in turn. First ask the patient where any tender areas are (examine these areas last of all and be particularly gentle there) and ask her to point to any specific lumps.

Examine the normal side first; ask the patient to place her hand behind her head on the side being examined (Fig. 5.4). Use gentle palpation with flattened fingers compressing the breast tissue against the chest wall and a rotating movement. Move around the breast, initially palpating superficially then deeper, to examine all four quadrants of the breast and the axillary tail.

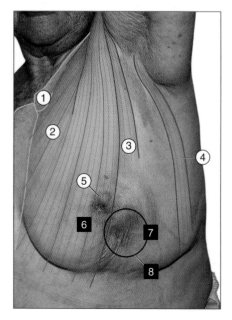

Fig. 5.3 Palpable breast lump.

① Clavicle
② Pectoralis major
③ Pectoralis minor
④ Latissimus dorsus
⑤ Areola
6 Indrawn nipple
7 Skin tethering
8 Site of cancer

Remember to be particularly careful with the tender breast and also examine behind the nipple/areolar regions. If the history has suggested a nipple discharge, ask the patient to squeeze the breast to produce discharge (and use a urinary dipstick to test for blood). If there is a lump, comment on its characteristics as follows:

- Size: ideally measured with callipers
- Shape: discrete lump(s) or diffuse swelling?
- Position: which breast?
  - which quadrant of the breast?
  - inner or outer aspect?
  - position on the clock face (Fig. 5.5)
- Fixation: tethering or fixation to the skin or underlying muscle
- Consistency: hard/craggy/soft/tender/fluctuant?
- Additional features: single or multiple?
  - axillary/cervical lymphadenopathy?
  - lumps in the contralateral breast?
  - previous scars/skin changes.

To test for fixation to the chest wall, the patient should tense her chest wall muscles while you try to move the lump. If the lump is

Fig. 5.4 Position of the patient for right breast examination.

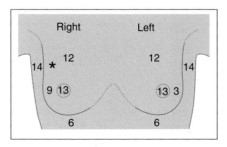

Fig. 5.5 Record the findings using positions of the clock (13 = central, 14 = axillary tail).

mobile when the patient is relaxed, but fixed when pectoralis major is tightened, then the tumour is tethered to the muscle.

Despite the inaccuracy of clinical examination in determining whether small axillary lymph nodes are involved with metastatic tumour, you still need to examine the regional lymph nodes. To examine for axillary lymph nodes, take the patient's left arm with yours, then, using your right hand, examine the four walls of the axilla (medial, lateral, anterior, posterior) and its apex for palpable lymph nodes. Note where the nodes are palpable, whether there are a few scattered ('shotty') nodes (the sort you may well be able to feel in your own axilla), or large or matted nodes (Fig. 5.6), and whether they are fixed to the surrounding structures. Whether or not you can feel any lymphadenopathy in the axilla, it is also mandatory to examine the infraclavicular, supraclavicular and cervical regions for lymphadenopathy, noting the presence of nodes as for the axilla.

Summary

Summarize the findings. Remember to comment on the following, even if negative.

Fig. 5.6 Clinical signs of breast cancer.

① Clavicle
② Pectoralis major
③ Pectoralis minor
④ Areola
5 Indrawn nipple
6 Skin tethering
7 Site of cancer
8 Cancer infiltrating skin
9 Node mass

HISTORY

- Age
- Length of time lump has been present
- Associated features, i.e. nipple discharge/Skin changes
- Menopausal status and points
- Family history.

FEATURES OF LUMP

- Size
- Shape/consistency
- Position
- Fixation.

AXILLARY/REGIONAL LYMPH NODES

- Palpable or not
- Matted or not.

For example, a summary of the case illustrated in Fig. 5.6 might be: 'A 60-year-old woman with a single, palpable 6 cm, hard, non-tender lump in the 10 o'clock position of the upper quadrant of the right breast, 3 cm from the areolar margin. Fixed to the deeper tissues and tethered to the skin with skin erythema. There are associated palpable matted 3 cm lymph nodes fixed to each other, and palpable in the medial wall of the axilla, though no supraclavicular or cervical lymphadenopathy.'

You may be asked if there is any other part of the patient that you wish to examine: this is to remind you to examine the contralateral breast for a second cancer (if you have not already done so) and the liver for metastatic disease. Examination of the abdomen for hepato-megaly can be part of the follow-up clinical examination of a patient with breast cancer, and should be mentioned to the examiner.

INVESTIGATIONS

After the examination, the next task is to establish whether or not this lump is a cancer. Current guidelines dictate 'triple modality' diagnostic criteria for a clinically suspicious lump: a cancer clinically, a cancer mammographically and a cancer on fine-needle aspiration cytology (or core biopsy) (Fig. 5.7).

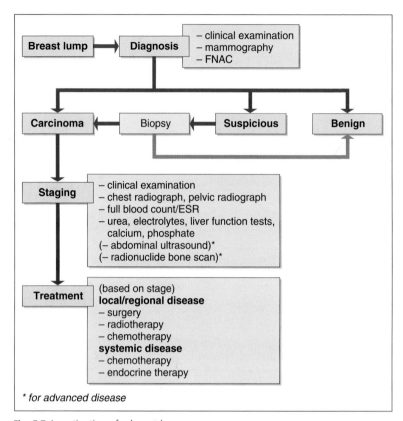

Fig. 5.7 Investigation of a breast lump.

KEY POINTS

- Diagnosis of a breast lump is by triple assessment:
  - clinical
  - radiological
  - cytopathology

Mammography

This is performed in two views on each breast: craniocaudal (up/down view) and oblique (showing the axillary tail of the breast, part of pectoralis major and the breast itself) (Fig. 5.8), and may be supplemented by additional views. Mammography may demonstrate normal architecture (with breast tissue of variable density, usually most dense in young

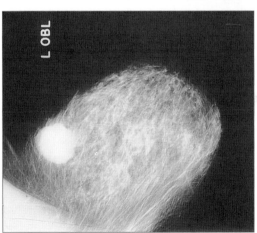

Fig. 5.8 Mammogram of left breast cancer.

① Pectoralis major   **2** Cancer   ③ Normal breast tissue women, distorted architecture, masses or (micro-)calcification. The two breasts are compared for differences in architecture. About 95% of breast cancers show up on mammography.

Breast ultrasonography

This is particularly useful in the under-35 age group, because mammography of dense breast tissue is difficult to interpret. Ultrasonography can be used to examine areas of lumpy breast, and may distinguish a common benign lump such as a fibroadenoma from a cancer by virtue of the outline of the lump and the acoustic shadow cast.

Fine needle aspiration cytology (FNAC)

This involves inserting a 21-gauge (blue) needle on a 10 ml syringe into the palpable area, and passing the needle to and fro through the area 10 or more times while gentle suction is applied using the syringe. The aspirate (which may be quite scanty) is then expressed on to glass slides, spread and either air-dried or fixed. A cytopathologist can subsequently examine the (stained) slides for cells, including breast cancer cells. In good hands (i.e. aspirator and cytopathologist), the diagnostic success rate is over 95%. FNAC can be performed either freehand (in the case of a palpable lump) or (for an impalpable breast lesion) using ultrasonography or stereotactic mammography guidance. Alternatively, or to confirm the diagnosis, core biopsies (2–3 mm in diameter) may be obtained under local anaesthetic.

Radiological tests

These include a chest radiograph (for lung metastases or pleural effusion, liver ultrasound scan (reserved for advanced cancers, in which liver metastases are more likely), plain radiographs of symptomatic bony areas and an isotope bone scan (for bone metastases).

Other investigations

These may include a full blood count (for anaemia, marrow infiltration, white count pre- and post-chemotherapy), erythrocyte sedimentation rate (may be raised in malignancy), levels of urea, electrolytes and creatinine (renal impairment may influence the choice and dosage of chemotherapy) and liver function tests (though a poor indicator of liver metastases).

Table 5.1 Staging of breast cancer

Tumours	T: cancer clinically <2 cm T2: cancer clinically 2–5 cm T3: cancer clinically >5 cm T4: cancer involving skin or chest wall
Nodes	N0: no regional node metastasis N1: metastasis to movable ipsilateral axillary nodes N2: metastasis to fixed ipsilateral axillary nodes
Metastasis	M0: no metastasis M1: distant metastasis

MANAGEMENT

On the basis of the diagnostic and clinical tests, the patient can be 'staged' according to the TNM (tumour, node, metastasis) system (Table 5.1) or as stages I, II, III, IV and the most suitable management of the individual patient can be decided. For patients with breast cancer, this may include surgery to the breast (lump or breast removal), surgery to the axilla (sentinel node biopsy, axillary node sampling or clearance), radiotherapy of the breast/chest wall and/or axillary tissues, endocrine therapy (e.g. tamoxifen, aromatase inhibitors), endocrine ablation (e.g. LHRH [luteinizing hormone-releasing hormone] analogues, oophorectomy) and chemotherapy (bolus or infusional; before surgery, or postoperatively as adjuvant therapy). Which therapy to give to whom (and when) is best addressed by a multidisciplinary team including surgeon, oncologist, pathologist and nurse counsellor.

TYPICAL CASES

Single breast lump*

HISTORY

A single breast lump is a common breast problem in the final surgical exam. In women aged under 30 years, a single breast lump is most likely to be benign (benign breast tissue or, if discrete, a fibroadenoma – Fig. 5.9), although it could be malignant. In the age range 30–45 years it is likely to be a cyst (see 'Multiple breast lumps') or carcinoma.

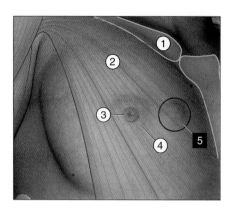

Fig. 5.9 Fibroadenoma.

① Clavicle
② Pectoralis major
③ Nipple
④ Areola
5 Fibroadenoma

Over 45 years of age, a single breast lump should be considered to be a breast cancer until proven otherwise (see Fig. 5.1).

Examination

Follow the examination plan described above. If the patient turns out to have a single breast lump that you suspect may be a cancer, discuss the possible management with the examiner as outlined above.

In a young woman, normal breast tissue may give the impression of a discrete lump, which should fade away after her menses. A truly discrete lump, which is usually very mobile (hence its name 'breast mouse'), is likely to be a fibroadenoma and more than one may be present in the breast.

Investigations

Clinical diagnosis should be backed up by mammography (in patients aged over 35 years), breast ultrasonography and FNAC. The importance of a fibroadenoma lies in distinguishing it from more sinister breast lumps; once the diagnosis of a fibroadenoma has been established, most of these lumps do not need to be removed, and remain static in size for some years. However, if a clinician harbours residual doubts about a diagnosis, or if the patient strongly requests excision of a lump, then the lump should be removed (under local or general anaesthetic). If a cancer is diagnosed, the staging investigations outlined above are used to decide whether breast conservation is practicable. In general, for breast conservation the tumour should be 4 cm or less in size, without skin or chest wall involvement, and the breast should be large enough to allow excision of the tumour and a rim of breast tissue without unduly distorting the breast.

Multiple breast lumps*

Multiple breast lumps in a patient in the exam are most likely to be breast cysts in a middle-aged woman. However, occasionally patients with benign lumpy breasts, multiple fibroadenomas or bilateral or multiple breast cancers may find their way into the exam.

HISTORY AND EXAMINATION

History taking and examination should be as outlined above. Women with breast cysts have often experienced them before. They appear as lumps that are smooth and usually non-tender, often in both breasts. They may appear to be single or multiple and either small or quite large, and may even distort the size and shape of the breasts quite considerably. Bilateral breast examination should be followed by examination of the axillary, infraclavicular/supraclavicular and cervical nodes. Figure 5.10 shows a 45-year-old woman with a 2.5 cm lump in the 9 o'clock position of the right breast.

There was a further lump in the 6 o'clock position of the left breast. The lumps are smooth in outline, non-tender and mobile.

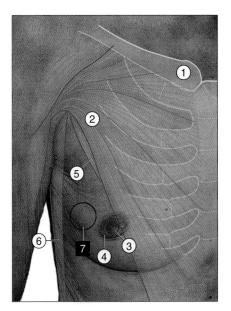

Fig. 5.10 Breast cyst.

① Clavicle
② Pectoralis major
③ Nipple
④ Areola
⑤ Pectoralis minor
⑥ Latissimus dorsi
7 Breast cyst

INVESTIGATIONS

Mammography (or preferably breast ultrasonography in a patient aged under 35 years) will reveal the well-circumscribed outline of a cyst, and should be used to help exclude any other impalpable breast pathology. Aspiration with a needle and syringe will confirm the diagnosis, and treat the cysts. The colour of the cystic fluid, which may be clear, opalescent or green through to almost black, and its volume (usually 5–20 ml, but occasionally up to 100 ml) are of little consequence. However, a bloody aspirate, a residual mass after aspiration or cysts that recur a third time after two aspirations 3 weeks apart may indicate an underlying cancer and such areas should be excised (Fig. 5.11). Patients with multiple cysts may decide to live with their cysts, asking for only particularly prominent lumps to be aspirated.

Post-mastectomy patient*

HISTORY

In addition to the basic breast history already outlined, patients who have undergone treatment for breast cancer may be asked what surgery

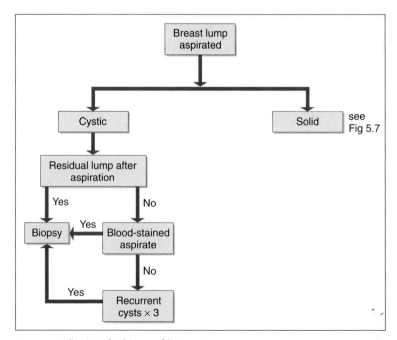

Fig. 5.11 Indications for biopsy of breast cyst.

they have had (particularly to the breast, axilla and abdomen), whether they have had radiotherapy (to the breast or chest wall alone or to the axilla also) and/or chemotherapy (before or after surgery, or both), and what medications they have had previously and are now taking, and for how long.

EXAMINATION

Inspect the chest and compare the two sides for scars: a mastectomy scar is usually transverse (Fig. 5.12), sometimes angling up into the axilla. Most mastectomy operations now leave the pectoralis major muscle in place (i.e. modified radical or Patey mastectomy) rather than involving radical mastectomy (with removal of pectoralis major). Look for the signs of radiotherapy: vascular telangiectasia of the skin in the field of irradiation, which may include the infra- or supraclavicular regions in addition to the chest wall. Diffuse skin thickening may also occur after radiotherapy, or the skin may appear thin, shiny and atrophic.

As a consequence of axillary node clearance and/or axillary radio-therapy or axillary nodal disease, some patients develop upper limb oedema which appears as mild to severe swelling of the hand, forearm

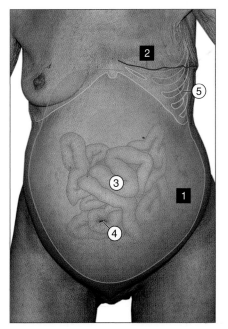

Fig. 5.12 Post-mastectomy patient.

1 Ascites
2 Mastectomy Scan
③ Small intestines
④ umbilicus
⑤ rbs

and/or upper arm. Remember to inspect the other breast (if present) for features of breast disease.

Palpation over the treated post-mastectomy chest wall should include feeling for any skin nodules (tumour metastases or buried sutures?) and up into the axilla for nodes or masses. The supraclavicular, infraclavicular and cervical nodes should also be palpated.

INVESTIGATIONS

Investigations performed routinely in post-mastectomy patients include annual mammography of the contralateral breast, to detect a second primary breast cancer (detected in 1–3% of patients per annum).

Breast-conservation patient**

HISTORY

Breast conservation is the term used to describe patients who have had a breast cancer removed (wide local excision) but in whom the remainder of the breast has been conserved (Fig. 5.13). Therefore, after asking the general breast history questions, you will need to ask patients who have undergone breast conservation treatment what surgery they have had to the breast (e.g. was the lumpectomy successful at the first excision?), axilla (e.g. were the lymph nodes sampled or cleared from the axilla?) and abdomen (e.g. was oophorectomy performed?). Many breast-conservation patients have adjuvant radiotherapy of the residual

Fig. 5.13 Breast-conservation patient.

breast (and axilla unless the nodes have been cleared) in case of microscopic residual disease, and adjuvant endocrine therapy (such as tamoxifen) or chemotherapy (particularly for premenopausal women with node involvement): you will need to ask about these aspects of the patient's treatment.

EXAMINATION

Inspect and compare the two breasts in terms of general size, shape and contour. Look for scars on the breast (from lumpectomy) and in the axilla (from node excision). After breast conservation there may be distortion of the appearance of the breast. There may also be signs of radiotherapy, particularly diffuse skin thickening. Remember to inspect both breasts thoroughly. Figure 5.13 shows a lumpectomy scar and an axillary scar (from an axillary node procedure). Look also for regional nodes (supraclavicular) and skin changes caused by radiotherapy.

Palpation over the treated breast should include the lumpectomy site (where there may be palpable scar tissue), the residual breast tissue (for further lumps) and then the axilla and the supraclavicular, infraclavicular and cervical nodes. Do not forget to examine the untreated breast.

Annual mammography of the treated breast and the contralateral side should be carried out, to detect recurrent disease or a second primary breast cancer. Long-term survival is no worse after wide local excision with radiotherapy than after mastectomy.

Gynaecomastia**

HISTORY

Gynaecomastia usually has one of three causes: physiological (in young men); induced by drugs (particularly cimetidine, or cardiac drugs including digoxin and spironolactone); or a systemic hormonal upset (particularly liver disease, hormonal therapy for prostate cancer, or testicular or pituitary tumours). Therefore, the history should include the patient's age and the timing of onset and duration of the swollen breast tissue. Is the gynaecomastia unilateral or bilateral? Is it tender or embarrassing? Ask about alcohol intake and drug history (with particular regard to cardiac or prostate cancer therapy), and whether the patient has had prostate surgery or noted a lump in a testicle.

EXAMINATION

Examination of the male breast should be performed as for the female breast: often, simple exposure of the torso with the patient sitting and then inspection will suggest the diagnosis of gynaecomastia. If the underlying cause of the gynaecomastia is hepatic, some of the many signs of liver disease may be visible. You are unlikely to be asked to examine a man with breast cancer, but remember that male breast cancer does exist. It usually presents in elderly men at a locally advanced stage (including skin infiltration and often nodal disease too).

Before palpation of the breast tissue, ask whether it is tender. Usually gynaecomastia is palpable as a firm retroareolar mass, although it may be to one side of the breast area. Palpate for axillary and cervical lymphadenopathy, and remember to check the contralateral side.

The examination of a man with gynaecomastia should include the testes, because gynaecomastia is a possible presentation of testicular cancer. You should mention this in the exam, but you are unlikely to be asked to perform testicular examination on such a patient. Similarly you should comment on other secondary sexual characteristics such as hair loss, testicular atrophy or voice changes.

INVESTIGATIONS

The investigation of gynaecomastia should be aimed at determining the nature of the lump (to exclude carcinoma) and excluding serious pathology elsewhere. FNAC can be used to confirm the diagnosis.

Ultrasonography of a testicular lump, radiological views of the pituitary fossa and/or serum prolactin level may all be suggested as suitable investigations. Investigations for liver disease (see Chapter 6) may be appropriate in a patient with other signs of hepatic disease.

TREATMENT

The two main methods of treatment are discontinuation of a medication responsible for the gynaecomastia (which should result in a reduction of the swelling) and surgical excision of the offending tissue (if the patient wishes).

Breast cancer metastasis***

Breast cancer may commonly metastasize, usually to bones, liver, lungs, pleurae, peritoneal cavity, brain or subcutaneous tissues. A patient with metastatic breast cancer may be used as a long case in surgical finals, or as a short case for the detection of ascites (Fig. 5.12), a palpable liver or a pleural effusion.

Nipple discharge***

Nipple discharge is a common symptom, usually physiological. You need to ask whether the discharge is from one nipple or both, whether it is from only one duct on the nipple, and what colour it is (clear [physiological]; milky as a result of galactorrhoea, greenish or cheesy as a result of duct ectasia, or brown or blood stained as a result of a duct papilloma or carcinoma).

The detection of blood in the discharge requires that you test for blood with a dipstick unless frank red blood is being emitted from the nipple. Clearly, there will be concern about a blood-stained discharge from a single duct, which may signify an underlying carcinoma. Other investigations, including mammography, should aim to exclude a cancer.

Nipple eczema***

Nipples that appear to be eczematous may be just that, but beware of Paget's disease of the nipple (breast carcinoma cells in the nipple skin), which can have an identical appearance. Thus, if a woman who is middle-aged or older, and has no skin problems elsewhere, presents with nipple eczema, you will need to exclude Paget's disease and an underlying carcinoma.

Breast abscess***

A breast abscess is usually so painful that the woman concerned is unlikely to consent to appearing in an exam. Breast abscesses occur in breast-feeding mothers and in smokers. You should look for the features of inflammation (hot, red, tender, swollen, loss of function). Resolution may be achieved by using antibiotics, aspiration of the pus under anti-biotic cover or open drainage. Be aware that an inflammatory carcinoma of the breast may present with all the appearances of an abscess.

Skin lesions***

Skin lesions (e.g. sebaceous cyst, papilloma, lipoma) may occur on the breast and adjacent chest wall.

KEY QUESTIONS

1. What questions would you ask a patient with breast symptoms?
2. How do you describe a breast cancer after clinical examination?
3. How would you diagnose a breast cancer?
4. What are the clinical features of a breast cancer on examination?
5. Where does breast cancer metastasize to?
6. What are the common diagnoses of a breast lump in a 30-year-old woman, a 40-year-old woman and a 70-year-old woman?
7. What features of previous breast cancer treatment might you see on the chest wall?

6

Abdomen

Abdominal examination forms one of the key parts of surgical finals. Students often worry about where to start in a short case when asked to 'examine the gastrointestinal system' which (confusingly) means start with the hands, examine the head and neck, look in the mouth and examine the chest wall *before* you approach the abdomen. On the other hand, when an examiner asks you to 'examine the abdomen' in surgical circles, he or she means exactly that! As the abdominal contents lie close to each other behind a sometimes substantial abdominal wall, it is useful to know the surface markings of abdominal organs (Figs 6.1 and 6.2).

KEY POINT

- The history (70%), examination (20%) and investigations (10%) contribute to the diagnosis of abdominal disorders

---

HISTORY

Some important general questions often get overlooked in considering the abdomen, but may point to the diagnosis, including the age, gender, occupation, social history (alcohol intake, smoking) and drug history (as a potential cause of abdominal symptoms, or taken to relieve abdominal symptoms). Family history may be important for a range of abdominal problems including colon cancer and inflammatory bowel disease.

Systemic manifestations of abdominal disease processes include loss of appetite, weight loss or weight gain (in kilograms or pounds, or measured by change in size of clothing or belt), nausea, pallor, jaundice, itch and bruising.

Systematic questions about the abdominal gastrointestinal tract should include the following.

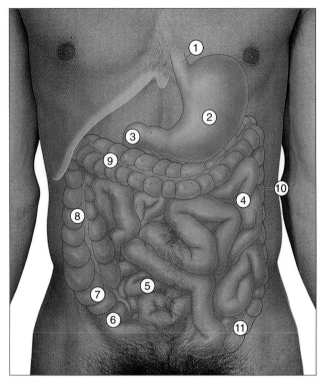

Fig. 6.1 Surface markings of the alimentary tract.

① Oesophagus   ⑤ Ileum   ⑨ Transverse colon
② Stomach   ⑥ Appendix   ⑩ Descending colon
③ Duodenum   ⑦ Caecum   ⑪ Sigmoid colon
④ Jejunum   ⑧ Ascending colon

MOUTH

Ask about ulcers or discomfort in the mouth, taste and salivary gland swelling.

SWALLOWING

If there is difficulty swallowing, ask about onset, duration and any progression from solids (often meat is the first problem noted) to liquids or even inability to swallow saliva.

Fig. 6.2 Surface markings of the abdominal viscera.

① Liver   ④ Pancreas   ⑦ Ureter
② Gallbladder   ⑤ Spleen   ⑧ Aorta
③ Duodenum   ⑥ Kidney   ⑨ Vena cava

VOMITING

What is its timing in relation to food ingestion? Is the food recognizable or partly/fully digested? What is the colour of the vomitus – opalescent fluid (pure gastric juice), brown (bile), green (proximal small bowel), feculent (distal small bowel)?

WATERBRASH

Ask if there is regurgitation of gastric contents into the oesophagus and pharynx.

INDIGESTION

Ask if there is a burning sensation in the epigastrium.

ABDOMINAL PAIN

This can be described in detail by a patient in response to the following questions and strongly suggests the likely diagnosis:

- When did the pain start?
- Where does it occur?
- When does it occur?
- Can the pain be described (sharp/dull/burning/gripping)?
- How often does the pain occur (periodicity)?
- Where does the pain radiate to?
- What are the aggravating factors?
- What are the relieving factors?
- What are the associated features?
- Have you ever had this pain before?

ABDOMINAL DISTENSION (BLOATING)

If this occurs, is it intermittent (and what is the periodicity) or progressive?

BOWEL HABIT

Has there been any change in bowel habit, increasing constipation or diarrhoea, either of which may be intermittent or progressive?

What are the consistency, colour, smell and features of the stool, and how has the stool changed recently? Does the stool flush away easily or with difficulty?

Has the patient noted any blood, mucus or pus passed per anus? If blood was noted was it fresh red blood or old dark blood, clots or liquid, mixed in with the stool or separate from the stool or on the toilet paper only? Did this occur once or on multiple occasions?

Is there any pain on defecation or any faecal or urinary incontinence? Have there been problems with itch, abscesses or fistulae in the area?

GYNAECOLOGICAL HISTORY

This should include the date of the last menstrual period, whether the patient is currently pregnant, the number of pregnancies and mode of delivery. Ask whether there is vaginal discharge, midcycle pain, pain at the time of menses, or intermenstrual or postmenopausal bleeding.

PAST MEDICAL HISTORY

The past medical history should include previous surgery and medical illnesses, and past drug use (prescribed and 'recreational'). History of jaundice, travel abroad, contact with farm or household animals, and sexual history may all be of relevance to abdominal diagnoses.

FAMILY HISTORY

Family history may be particularly relevant for colorectal cancer, inflammatory bowel disease and rare conditions such as familial adenomatous polyposis, Peutz–Jeghers syndrome or hereditary haemorrhagic telangiectasia.

EXAMINATION

Remember that, in a short case, the examiner will be watching to see how you conduct an examination of the patient, and this is perhaps even more important than what you find. Wash your hands. Approach the patient so as to be at his or her right-hand side. Then introduce yourself – this is a good way to start, because it breaks the ice.

Abdominal examination may be facilitated by first examining other parts of the body (hands, head and neck, lower limbs) for systemic signs of intra-abdominal conditions. Look for the following:

- Hands: finger clubbing, palmar erythema, Dupuytren's contracture, leukonychia
- Head and neck: jaundice of the sclera or pallor of the conjunctivae, spider naevi, telangiectasia, perioral pigmented spots
- Chest: gynaecomastia, missing breast (for intra-abdominal metastases from breast cancer)
- Lower limbs: peripheral oedema, scratch marks, bruising, erythema nodosum.

Exposure/positioning

Position the patient lying comfortably on his back, head resting on one pillow, hands by the sides, legs uncrossed and exposed from nipple to groin, so that you can see and subsequently feel the abdomen.

Inspection

Close inspection can give you many clues as to what you may find during subsequent palpation, percussion and auscultation. Watch for movement (or lack of movement as a result of abdominal pain) on respiration, visible peristalsis, abdominal masses or asymmetry.

Look for surgical scars (Fig. 6.3), not only on the anterior abdominal wall but also in the flanks and the groin (perhaps hidden by hair or fat), at the umbilicus and on the chest wall. Small surgical scars (from laparoscopy) and skin crease incisions can heal remarkably well.

Look for obvious features such as a stoma, which may be hidden by a stoma bag, fistulae, masses and skin changes (distended veins, skin lesions, bruising, erythema, ab igne).

If there is a stoma (Fig. 6.4 and Table 6.1) ask yourself:

- Where is it in the abdomen?
- Does it protrude from or is it flush with the abdominal surface?

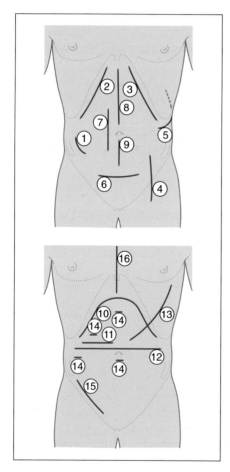

Fig. 6.3 Abdominal scars.

① Lanz (appendix)
② Kocher's (hepatobiliary)
③ Left subcostal (spleen)
④ Vascular
⑤ Nephrectomy (extraperitoneal)
⑥ Pfannenstiel (gynaecology or caesarean section)
⑦ Right paramedian
⑧ Upper midline
⑨ Lower midline
⑩ Roof-top (pancreatobiliary)
⑪ Tranvserse (gallbladder, colectomy)
⑫ Transverse (abdominal aortic aneurysm, colonic surgery)
⑬ Thoracoabdominal (extending over left thorax; gastro-oesophageal surgery)
⑭ Laparoscopic port sites (for laparoscopic cholecystectomy)
⑮ Inguinal hernia
⑯ Sternotomy

Fig. 6.4 Abdominal stoma.

1 Ileostomy or urostomy (spout)

2 Double-barrel (loop) colostomy

3 End-colostomy

4 Mucous fistula

Table 6.1 Features of stoma

Types of stoma		Features
Colostomy		
	End	Mucosa flush with skin, produces formed faeces
	Loop	Two lumens (like double-barrelled shotgun), one producing solid stool
	Mucous fistula	Mucosa flush with skin but only small amounts of mucus
Ileostomy		
	End	Stoma protrudes 3–4 cm beyond skin surface, liquid stool
	Loop	Two lumina, one producing liquid stool
Urostomy	Like end-ileostomy, but producing cloudy (as a result of ileal mucus) urine	

- What is it producing (solids, liquid stool or urine)?
- Is there one opening or two?

Remember that a colostomy is usually (but not exclusively) in the LIF (left iliac fossa) (Fig. 6.5), should lie flush with the skin and when mature produces a formed stool. An ileostomy should protrude as a 2–3 cm spout (Fig. 6.6) to protect the surrounding skin, is often located in the RIF (right iliac fossa) and produces liquid stool, sometimes in

Fig. 6.5 End colostomy.

1 Colostomy   ③ Descending colon   ⑤ Anterosuperior iliac spine
2 Laparotomy scar   ④ Rectus sheath   ⑥ Inguinal ligament

Fig. 6.6 Ileostomy.

1 Ileostomy   ③ Intra-abdominal ileum   ⑤ Anterosuperior iliac spine
2 Laparatomy scar   ④ Rectus sheath   ⑥ Inguinal ligament

considerable amounts. Either a colostomy or an ileostomy can be an end-stoma or a loop of bowel brought to the surface as a loop stoma (or double-barrel stoma). To add to the potential confusion, end-stomas and loop stomas produce bowel content whereas a mucous fistula (usually at end of sigmoid colon) does not, being one end of a defunctioned length of bowel. A urostomy may look similar to the spout of an ileostomy, but involves an isolated length of ileum into which the ureters have been plumbed, which acts as a conduit for urine. A urostomy produces urine, recognizable by its colour, although often a little cloudy as a result of the ileal mucus production.

The complications of an abdominal stoma include retraction, prolapse, stenosis, parastomal hernia and dehydration/electrolyte imbalance.

If an abdominal mass is apparent, ask the patient to raise his head off the pillow to try to determine whether the mass is intra-abdominal (the mass disappears) or on the surface of the abdominal wall (the mass persists). Ask the patient to give a big cough to emphasize any hernias and look to see whether he or she winces because of abdominal pain when coughing or moving.

Palpation

Ask the patient's permission to examine (palpate) his or her abdomen, and before you start ensure that both of you are in a comfortable position. Kneeling beside the bed at the patient's right-hand side (not sitting on the bed) is one ideal position in the eyes of some examiners. Before you touch the patient ask 'Are you sore anywhere?' and, if so ask him or her to point out the tender areas. Leave touching any painful areas until last. Watch the patient's face (to see if you are causing discomfort) and gently palpate, rotating between the four quadrants of the abdomen. Follow this with deeper (but still gentle) palpation. By now you should have identified and delineated any obvious masses. If you feel a mass, make sure that you define its extent (this may be difficult for a mass arising from the pelvis, in which case you should say so). What is the size of the mass? Is it possible to indent the mass (faeces will indent)? Can you ballott the mass (kidney)? Is it expansile (i.e. an aneurysm)?

PALPATION FOR SPECIFIC FEATURES

The liver

To feel for the edge of the liver, start in the RIF and palpate towards the right costal margin, using the tips of your fingers gently applied to the abdominal wall. The edge of the liver, if palpable, will move inferiorly with each deep inspiration, and will meet your fingers. Be careful to ensure that if you feel a mass you cannot insinuate your fingers between this and the costal margin – if this is possible it is not the liver that you are feeling! You can then define the lower border of the liver and state how far (in centimetres) it lies below the costal margin. You cannot state that the liver is enlarged until you have defined (by percussion) its upper border (normally in the midclavicular line of the fourth intercostal space). If in doubt as to the position of the lower border of the liver, listen with your stethoscope over the presumed liver edge and use your index finger gently to scratch the skin along a line perpendicular to the presumed edge and extending across it (from the skin overlying the liver to that over the rest of the abdomen). There is a change in the quality and pitch of the sound heard as you pass from solid (liver) to hollow organ (intestines). Having felt a liver edge, state whether the liver is tender or not. Is the liver smooth (usually benign) or craggy (often neoplastic), soft or firm, pulsatile (suggesting tricuspid regurgitation) or hard (tumour)? As you examine, sneak a look for other general signs that might lead you to likely causes of hepatomegaly (see below).

KEY POINTS

- Start in (R) iliac fossa and palpate towards (R) costal margin
- Feel whole length of liver border
- Comment on tenderness and consistency of liver

The spleen

Again start in the RIF (not the LIF or you may miss a large spleen), palpating as for a liver edge but this time towards the left costal margin. If you cannot feel the spleen, roll the patient towards you (to lie on the right side) and feel under the left costal margin on deep inspiration. Comment on whether it is possible to palpate 'above' the spleen (i.e. between the spleen and the costal margin); this should not be possible in the case of the spleen, but should be possible in the case of an enlarged left kidney. The spleen typically has a palpable notch that may distinguish it from other masses.

KEY POINTS

- Start in (R) iliac fossa feeling towards (L) costal margin
- Consider rotation of the patient if spleen difficult to feel

The kidneys

Using bimanual palpation on inspiration, try to palpate each kidney in turn. Place the flat of one hand behind the patient, under the loin, and the other hand on the upper quadrant of the same side. On deep inspiration, a normal kidney may just be palpable in a thin person (particularly on the right-hand side, where it lies a little lower than on the left), descending to meet your anterior hand. You may also try to ballott the kidney with a sharp push from the posterior hand, pressing the kidney towards your other (anterior) hand. Even large kidneys (which are usually polycystic if really big) should not stop you from 'getting above' the kidney under the ribcage, which should not be possible in the case of the liver or spleen. If you percuss over an enlarged kidney, the note is often resonant because there will be overlying bowel gas – another means of determining whether the mass that you are feeling is really a kidney.

A word of caution: a transplanted kidney is usually placed in the RIF (where the renal artery and vein can be readily connected to the iliac vessels, and the ureter to the bladder). It is readily palpable, as a smooth subcutaneous mass beneath a scar very like a long appendectomy scar – a sneaky trick putting it there, but if you know it's a possibility, forewarned is forearmed.

KEY POINTS

- Kidneys are ballottable
- You should be able to get your hand above the (L) kidney
- Percussion over either kidney is generally resonant

Aortic aneurysm

An abdominal aortic aneurysm (AAA) can be missed unless you remember to palpate specifically for an expansile mass adjacent to the umbilicus. Place your index fingers on either side of the line of the aorta, gently pressing to feel the sensation of the fingers being pushed apart. It is difficult to comment on the size of an abdominal aortic aneurysm without ultrasonography, but in a thin person an aneurysm may be readily palpable.

KEY POINTS

- An abdominal aortic aneurysm is truly expansile
- This will differentiate if from transmitted pulsation via an overlying mass

Percussion

Percuss all four quadrants of the abdomen. Don't press too hard when trying to percuss, and make sure your fingernails are not so long as to leave your hand sore. Percuss the margins of any masses that you have already identified. Is the mass tympanic or solid? Percuss the upper and lower borders of the liver and spleen, and the upper border of the bladder or uterus (occasionally a pregnant woman finds her way into finals).

Shifting dullness caused by ascites (Fig. 6.7) is often easier to demonstrate by percussion than by demonstrating a fluid thrill: successive percussion of your finger placed over the patient's flank, parallel to the spine, will delineate the fluid–air interface. Keep your finger over a place that has been dull to percussion as the patient rolls on to his or her side, then percuss again – if the dull note has become resonant as fluid has shifted elsewhere in the abdomen, shifting dullness has been demonstrated.

The possible cause for the ascites may be apparent on examination (Fig. 6.7).

Fig. 6.7 Malignant ascites from metastatic breast cancer.

1 Distended abdomen (fluid, dull to percussion)

2 Mastectomy scar

③ Bowel (resonant to percussion)

④ Umbilicus

⑤ Ribs

Auscultation

Using the diaphragm of the stethoscope, listen for bowel sounds (frequency, pitch, isolated/runs) over the abdomen, and if appropriate over any hernia. Runs of frequent, high-pitched bowel sounds can be heard when the bowel is obstructed. If the bowel sounds are scanty or absent (make sure that you listen for long enough), ileus or peritonitis is indicated.

Remember to listen for a hepatic bruit (suggesting hepatoma). If necessary, auscultate for the edge of the liver using the 'scratch' test described above. With the patient sitting, listen in the renal angle for a renal artery bruit posteriorly and for femoral artery bruits in the groin.

To seek a succussion splash (if you suspect gastric outflow obstruction), gently shake the supine patient from side to side then hold him or her still and listen. (You can sometimes hear your own succussion splash if you move around actively after a meal.)

Further examination

Finally, state that you would normally proceed to perform a digital rectal examination of every patient. It is usually said that there can be only two reasons for not doing so: either the patient has no anus (e.g. after abdominoperineal excision of the rectum) or you have no fingers. In an exam there is a third reason – the fact that it is an exam, and patients would not participate if they thought that they would have to undergo multiple rectal examinations. Vaginal examination should also be mentioned if this would be appropriate, but similarly you will not be expected to perform this on a patient in the exam.

However, with modern plastic models, in an OSCE you may be asked to perform a rectal or vaginal examination. State to the examiner that you would ask the patient's permission and require a chaperone.

Rectal examination using a gloved and lubricated finger will allow you to describe the sphincter tone, palpate the prostate in males (size, smooth/craggy, whether tender), and palpate the cervix in females (whether tender). Feel the rectal mucosa for any abnormalities and obtain a sample of faeces for occult blood testing.

Vaginal examination using two gloved lubricated fingers may be appropriate to palpate the gynaecological organs.

You must not forget that a basic abdominal examination should include testing a urine sample (for protein, blood and glucose as a minimum) and testing stool for faecal occult blood. You may be provided with a patient's urine sample to test in the exam.

Investigations

As the list of investigations for abdominal symptoms is extensive, decide what is needed to define the pathology going from least invasive (e.g. urinalysis) to more specialist tests (e.g. endoscopy) as appropriate. The following investigations may also be useful:

- Urine testing for pH, specific gravity, blood, protein, urobilinogen
- Pregnancy testing of urine (for β-hCG – human β-chorionic gonadotrophin)
- Faecal occult blood testing
- Haematology: haemoglobin, mean corpuscular volume (MCV), white cell count (WCC) with differential count, blood film, vitamin B_{12}, folate, international normalized ratio (INR), partial thromboplastin time – kaolin (PTTK), supplementary tests of the clotting cascade
- Erythrocyte sedimentation rate (ESR), plasma viscosity and C-reactive protein (CRP)
- Biochemistry: urea, sodium, potassium, chloride, creatinine, liver function tests (LFTs), amylase, serum tumour markers (CEA [carcinoembryonic antigen], CA-125, CA-153)
- Arterial blood gases: Po_2, Pco_2, bicarbonate, hydrogen ion, base excess
- Radiology (discussed in more detail below): plain erect chest and supine abdominal radiographs, ultrasonography, single- or double-contrast radiology, intravenous urogram, isotope renal scan, CT (with contrast), MRI, interventional techniques including percutaneous transhepatic cholangiography, angiography
- Endoscopy (with biopsy where appropriate): upper gastrointestinal endoscopy, endoscopic ultrasonography, enteroscopy, endoscopic retrograde cholangiopancreatography (ERCP), proctoscopy, rigid or flexible sigmoidoscopy, colonoscopy
- Laparoscopy (with peritoneal lavage or biopsy), laparoscopic ultrasonography
- Biopsy by fine needle, core or open incisional/excisional techniques.

ABDOMINAL RADIOLOGY

Abdominal radiographs of one sort or another are the most frequently encountered films in surgical finals. Similar to chest radiographs, they often have more than one abnormality and respond well to the thought 'Don't panic, I *can* work through this radiograph systematically, and detect the abnormalities'.

1. Check that the film is correctly oriented and on a well-lit viewing box.
2. Check the patient's name, and date of birth if it is visible.
3. Decide what sort of film you are examining. Is it a plain radiograph or has contrast been introduced into the patient? If there is contrast, is it inside the bowel (upper gastrointestinal tract, small bowel, colon) or inside another structure (biliary tree, vascular tree)? For gastrointestinal tract contrast examinations, is this a single-contrast study (i.e. a contrast agent such as barium) or a double-contrast study (e.g. barium + air, to give enhanced mucosal detail)? A CT scan or MRI series can find its way to exams. The examiner should ask you to look at one or two sections in particular. At first, CT scans and MR images can be really intimidating, but go through the same systematic process and you will at least detect the main abnormality.
4. Is there a gross abnormality?
5. Proceed to describe the film systematically:
   - hollow viscera (stomach/intestines, bowel gas pattern)
   - solid viscera (kidneys/liver outline, gas in the biliary tree)
   - vascular structures (calcification in the wall)
   - bony structures:
     - pelvic bones (contour and consistency)
     - thoracic/lumbar/sacral spine
     - ribs
     - femoral heads
   - subcutaneous tissues (lower chest, abdomen, pelvis).
6. Take a final look and draw your thoughts together.
7. Summarize what you can see.

In the rest of this chapter there are illustrative plain radiographs, CT scans and contrast studies; use the scheme to approach each radiograph.

TYPICAL CASES

Abdominal mass*

An abdominal mass is among the most common problems to be presented to you in the surgical exams. Most abdominal masses will be intra-abdominal, although masses may also indicate abdominal wall lesions such as a lipoma, a rectus muscle haematoma or a rare abdominal wall tumour. A lump within the abdominal wall is still palpable when the abdominal wall is tensed (e.g. when the patient lifts the head off the pillow), but an intra-abdominal mass is not.

KEY POINTS

- The patient's age and history and the position of an abdominal mass suggest the likely diagnosis
- The diagnosis should be confirmed by appropriate investigation

HISTORY

Remember to ask about gastrointestinal, urinary and gynaecological symptoms. The past medical history and, particularly, a history of surgical operations can be most helpful in suggesting the diagnosis.

EXAMINATION

Follow the scheme of exposure/positioning, inspection, palpation, percussion and auscultation, bearing in mind the anatomical structures present in each area and the possible causes of a palpable mass in each region. An abdominal mass is typically inflammatory or neoplastic. Figure 6.8 summarizes the possible locations and causes of abdominal

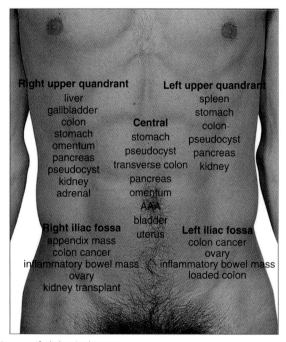

Fig. 6.8 Causes of abdominal masses.

masses. Remember that intra-abdominal lymph nodes and rare conditions such as a mesenteric cyst (a smooth swelling that is very mobile) may occur in any region of the abdomen. Your examiners will be more interested in your approach to the patient and their problem than necessarily the correct diagnosis.

Jaundice*

Icteric patients are surprisingly common on surgical wards, and in a surgical context their jaundice usually has a posthepatic cause. Prehepatic and hepatic jaundice are usually medical conditions, but should form part of your differential diagnosis in all jaundiced patients. Causes of jaundice to remember include:

- Prehepatic:
    - transfusion reactions
    - haemolysis secondary to sepsis or haematological disease
- Hepatic:
    - hepatitis (e.g. viral hepatitis A, B, C)
    - cirrhosis
    - drugs
- Posthepatic:
    - biliary obstruction caused by gallstones
    - primary cancer (pancreas, cholangiocarcinoma, ampullary carcinoma)
    - metastatic carcinoma of the liver
    - secondary carcinoma (e.g. of portal nodes)
    - sclerosing cholangitis.
    - benign biliary structures.

KEY POINTS

- Jaundice is usually posthepatic in surgical finals
- Ultrasonography is the single most useful investigation in determining whether this is the case

---

HISTORY

Remember to ask about fever, itch, bruising, dark urine, pale stools and other bowel symptoms (including those of inflammatory bowel disease). Ask about the timing of the onset of the jaundice, and whether it is progressive or intermittent and/or associated with abdominal or back pain. Patients with viral hepatitis often give a history of prodromal symptoms occurring before becoming frankly icteric. A history of travel abroad, blood transfusion, infectious contacts, tattoos, relevant occupation, alcohol or drugs (whether prescribed or not), or a family history (e.g. haemolytic) may lead you to a diagnosis. Common causes of hepatomegaly include cardiac failure, metastatic cancer or infection, so a past history of medical conditions or surgical resection for cancer may be significant.

EXAMINATION

With the patient lying comfortably, with one pillow and exposed from nipple to groin, inspect for the depth of jaundice, associated scratch marks (caused by pruritus), pallor, bruising, nutritional state and stigmata of chronic liver disease. These stigmata include spider naevi, palmar erythema, Dupuytren's contracture, bruising, flapping tremor, cerebral impairment, testicular atrophy, gynaecomastia, sparse body hair, peripheral oedema and caput medusae (a lot to spot at one glance!).

Palpate for lymphadenopathy in the neck, and for hepatomegaly, splenomegaly and testicular atrophy. Courvoisier's law is a common topic in surgical finals. In essence, it states that, if the gallbladder is palpable in a jaundiced patient, the jaundice is not likely to be caused by gallstones. This law is not absolute and relies on the finding that gallbladders containing stones are usually small and shrunken (and therefore impalpable), whereas gallbladder (and bile duct) distension may result from common bile duct obstruction, caused by, for example, a pancreatic carcinoma (hence the gallbladder is palpable where the ninth costal cartilage meets the costal margin).

Percuss for ascites (shifting dullness) and auscultate for a hepatic bruit.

An examination is theoretically incomplete without a rectal examination (for palpable tumour and occult or obvious blood) and urine testing. Testing the urine can enable you to distinguish between haemolytic jaundice (no bilirubin in the urine) and obstructive jaundice (water-soluble conjugated bilirubin in the urine, but no urobilinogen, as a result of interruption of the enterohepatic circulation).

INVESTIGATION

Investigations are summarized in Fig. 6.9.

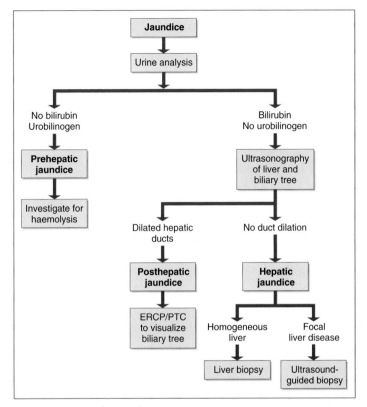

Fig. 6.9 Investigations for jaundice.

Urine test

Test for bilirubin and urobilinogen.

Basic haematology

Basic haematology, including coagulation and blood biochemistry should be performed to detect anaemia, raised WCC (in cholangitis), and raised platelet count (in splenic infarction resulting from splenic vein obstruction). Look at the levels of urea and electrolytes (beware of renal failure with jaundice, which is a lethal combination). Serum sodium may be low in cirrhosis.

Liver function tests

Alkaline phosphatase (ALP) and bilirubin levels are raised disproportionately compared with those of ALT (alanine aminotransferase) and GGT (γ-glutamyl transferase) in obstructive jaundice (Table 6.2). ALT levels are particularly high in hepatic forms of jaundice, but with prolonged jaundice the distinction becomes less clear. Albumin levels can be low in chronic liver disease (<30 g/l – severe; <20 g/l – bad news). Clotting may be abnormal, reflecting poor synthetic function, and will need correction before ERCP (see below) or surgery using vitamin K or, in emergency, blood products.

Radiology

Ultrasonography is useful for investigating gallstones (Fig. 6.10), liver size and texture, hepatic lesions >1 cm in size, dilated bile ducts (>6 mm in the case of the common bile duct), ascites and splenomegaly. However, its usefulness is severely limited by obesity and gaseous distension of the bowel (hence patients fast before scanning). A CT scan may provide the same information: it is less useful for investigating gallstones, but may be better for visualizing the pancreas, smaller hepatic lesions (Fig. 6.11), portal anatomy and blood flow (on dynamic scan).

Special tests

ERCP, performed with a side-viewing endoscope, is ideal for examining the ampulla, pancreatic duct and biliary tree. Percutaneous transhepatic cholangiography (PTC) is useful if the biliary tree is dilated or if

Table 6.2 Liver function tests in a jaundiced patient

Jaundice type	Test	Result
Hepatic jaundice	Bilirubin	↑↑↑
	ALT	↑↑↑
	GGT	↑↑↑
	ALP	↑
Obstructive jaundice	Bilirubin	↑↑↑
	ALT	↑
	GGT	↑
	ALP	↑↑↑

ALP, alkaline phosphatase; ALT, alanine aminotransferase; GGT, γ-glutamyl transferase.

Fig. 6.10 Ultrasound appearance in gallstone disease.

1 Gallstones   **2** Acoustic shadow   **3** Gallbladder

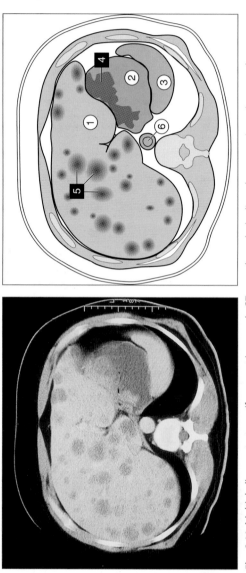

Fig. 6.11 Multiple liver metastases (from gastric cancer). CT scan through the liver demonstrating primary and metastatic gastric cancer.

① Liver   ② Stomach   ③ Spleen   ④ Gastric cancer   ⑤ Multiple liver metastases   ⑥ Aorta

ERCP is not possible (either not available or as a result of a technical failure, e.g. because of a previous Polya gastrectomy). Liver biopsy and/or laparoscopy, with or without laparoscopic ultrasonography, may also contribute to the diagnosis. Note the advent of novel non-invasive imaging techniques, such as endoscopic ultrasonography and MR cholangiography, which may surpass ERCP and PTC as ways of imaging the biliary tree.

MANAGEMENT

In addition to being asked about the diagnostic pathway in icteric patients, you may be asked about the problems that occur when such patients are operated upon. These problems may be related to haemostasis, fluid and electrolyte balance and renal failure, and/or malnutrition and immunosuppression, leading to poor wound healing and increased risk of infection.

Ascites*

The causes of ascites in patients likely to appear in surgical finals include cirrhosis (patients may also show signs of portal hypertension, such as splenomegaly or prominent abdominal wall veins), malignancy (particularly gastrointestinal, ovarian or breast cancers, Fig. 6.7), pancreatic ascites (secondary to pancreatitis with a high amylase level in the fluid), thrombosis of the portal vein after pancreatitis (may also lead to portal hypertension), hypoalbuminaemia (e.g. resulting from malnutrition, cirrhosis, cachexia in cancer), or obstruction/occlusion of the inferior vena cava or hepatic veins (known as Budd–Chiari syndrome in the latter case). Ascites may also be associated with pleural effusions or peripheral oedema.

KEY POINTS

- Shifting dullness on clinical examination, confirmed by ultrasonography

HISTORY

Remember that the causes of abdominal distension can be summarized as the five 'Fs': flatus, fluid (ascites), faeces, fetus and fat. When exploring the patient's history, include questions on conditions that predispose to ascites such as malignancy, alcoholic cirrhosis, pancreatitis and cardiac failure.

EXAMINATION

With the patient adequately exposed and in the correct position, inspect for signs of chronic liver disease (in addition to ascites), including: palmar erythema; Dupuytren's contracture; spider naevi; flapping tremor; testicular atrophy; gynaecomastia; peripheral oedema; hepatosplenomegaly; and caput medusae.

Test for shifting dullness (diagnostic of ascites) by percussion as outlined above. Confirmation of ascites can be obtained by looking for a fluid thrill – this requires an additional hand, and it is customary to ask the examiner for the use of his or her hand.

INVESTIGATIONS

- Serum albumin, sodium and potassium levels are of particular importance.
- Ultrasonography will demonstrate the ascitic fluid.
- A diagnostic tap of the ascites (using an 18-gauge needle/syringe into the RIF or LIF) can be used for the protein content, amylase level, cytology and bacteriology of the ascitic fluid.
- Upper gastrointestinal endoscopy should be considered in patients with portal hypertension, to detect the presence of oesophageal varices.

Hepatomegaly*

The three most common causes of *apparent* hepatomegaly are: a normal but palpable lower border of the liver (hence the importance of percussion to identify the upper border); cardiac failure; and metastatic disease involving the liver.

KEY POINTS

- Neoplastic, cardiac and infective causes
- Blood and radiological diagnosis

HISTORY

Remember the cardiac, neoplastic (primary or metastatic) and infective causes of hepatomegaly.

EXAMINATION

Inspect for signs of generalized liver disease, malignancy and cardiac failure.

Remember to define both the upper border of the liver (by percussion, in the fourth intercostal space in the midclavicular line) and the lower border (by palpation, percussion and/or the 'scratch' test). Ask yourself whether the edge of the liver is smooth/irregular, firm/soft, tender (e.g. in hepatitis, congestive cardiac failure) or pulsatile (e.g. with tricuspid regurgitation), and whether there is an audible bruit (e.g. with hepatoma). Examine for splenomegaly (see below).

INVESTIGATIONS

To supplement the routine haematological and biochemical investigations, the blood should be tested for AFP (α-fetoprotein, suggesting hepatoma) and carcinoembryonic antigen (CEA, suggesting colonic liver metastases).

An ultrasound scan, CT scan (see Fig. 6.11) and, if required, liver biopsy and laparoscopy should be used to establish the diagnosis.

Dysphagia*

Patients with dysphagia make a good long case. They are often elderly, and may have other disease states in addition to that causing the dysphagia. You must remember that dysphagia is always assumed to be the result of a significant pathology – there may be: oral/pharyngeal causes (unlikely to appear in surgical finals) or oesophageal causes, which may be intraluminal, mural (e.g. carcinoma, benign stricture, scleroderma), extramural (e.g. goitre, nodes, lung cancer) or neurological/functional.

KEY POINTS

- Usually the result of a disorder within the wall of the oesophagus (carcinoma or peptic stricture)
- Determine the severity of dysphagia and over what timescale it has been present
- Upper endoscopy is the key to identifying surgical causes of dysphagia

HISTORY

It is essential, first to grade dysphagia and, second, to determine whether it is progressive – if so, over what timescale. Find out if the patient can swallow solids, semisolids and liquids or has trouble with his or her own saliva (absolute dysphagia). Is this constant and progressive (often a tumour), constant but static (often a benign stricture) or intermittent (functional causes)? It is important to ask about weight loss, regurgitation and aspiration. If the patient is not sure about weight loss ask about how well (or not) their clothes fit.

The history should also include a full gastrointestinal enquiry. Remember to ask about medications (particularly NSAIDs [non-steroidal anti-inflammatory drugs], drugs for the treatment of ulcers or reflux, and iron).

A general medical history is important in assessing fitness for surgical treatment – many patients have cardiorespiratory diseases. Squamous oesophageal cancer affects the middle third of the oesophagus and is strongly linked to tobacco and alcohol usage. Lower oesophageal cancer (especially that occurring in Barrett's metaplastic oesophagus) is usually an adenocarcinoma and is associated with gastro-oesophageal reflux.

EXAMINATION

On inspection, is the general impression one of a well-nourished individual or is the patient cachectic, pale or jaundiced? Are there any signs of systemic disease, including rare conditions such as scleroderma?

Include in the examination the hands (for signs of, for example, loss of muscle mass, anaemia, scleroderma), then the head and neck (for systemic signs of malignant disease, particularly lymphadenopathy). Examine the chest, particularly for signs of lobar consolidation (caused by aspiration) and for pleural effusion (secondary to consolidation or malignancy). Examine the abdomen for an upper abdominal mass (carcinoma of the gastro-oesophageal junction commonly presents with dysphagia) and for hepatomegaly (e.g. caused by malignant disease).

INVESTIGATION

Investigations should include a full blood count (FBC), to detect anaemia in particular (e.g. caused by oesophagitis or carcinoma of the upper gastrointestinal tract, or associated with an oesophageal web). Blood biochemistry (to detect, for example, electrolyte disturbances, hypoalbuminaemia) and LFTs should also be carried out.

A chest radiograph (PA – posteroanterior) supplemented by a lateral film is useful, in order to look for hilar masses (e.g. hilar nodes, bronchogenic carcinoma) causing dysphagia. A barium swallow (to outline the oesophagus – Fig. 6.12) and meal (to examine the stomach) should be used to look for mucosal irregularity and abnormal contours. Ultrasonography may be useful for examining the liver and upper abdominal masses.

Upper gastrointestinal endoscopy (which some would contend should be carried out after a barium swallow has excluded a high obstructing oesophageal lesion) has the advantage that the mucosa can be directly visualized, and brushings or biopsies can be taken to investigate oesophagitis, Barrett's oesophagus, neoplasms (Figs 6.13 and 6.14) or candidal infection. Upper endoscopy can also be used therapeutically, and dilatation of a stricture or intubation of a neoplastic stricture using a stent may restore the ability to swallow fluids and food.

Abdominal pain*

Patients with abdominal pain make great exam subjects from the examiners' point of view, because they can lead to discussion of so many different facets of surgery and medicine.

Fig. 6.12 Barium swallow showing oeseophageal cancer.

1 Dilated oesophagus   ③ Stomach
2 Cancer   ④ Peristaltic wave   ⑤ Arch of aorta

Fig. 6.13 Obstructing oesophageal adenocarcinoma.

1 Cancer
② Lumen

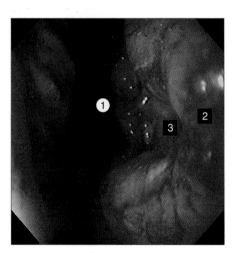

Fig. 6.14 Endoscopic view of ulcerated gastric cancer.

① Endoscope
2 Cancer
3 Ulcerated cancer

HISTORY

The history is all important in determining the likely cause of the abdominal pain. After a thorough history has been taken, you will be able to produce a differential diagnosis for the cause of the pain in most patients.

The age and gender of the patient form a good starting point for the determination of the likely disease processes going on. Remember the 10 features of pain:

1. Site (ask the patient to point with one finger; has the site of pain changed?)
2. Severity (compared with previous experiences)
3. Characteristics (e.g. sharp, burning, gnawing, dull)
4. Radiation (e.g. to back, around abdominal wall, into groin)
5. Onset (e.g. sudden, gradual, time of day)
6. Periodicity (over minutes, hours)
7. Relieving factors (e.g. movement, vomiting, lying still, leaning forwards)
8. Exacerbating factors (e.g. movement, drinking fluids)
9. Associated features (e.g. nausea, vomiting, changes in the colour of urine, stool or skin)
10. Previous episodes (hours/days/weeks/years ago; more/less severe; diagnosis then?).

This information will help to direct you to which system is involved, but do not forget to complete the history and systematic enquiry – there may be important features, such as past medical illnesses, previous operations, previous and current medications or medical conditions (e.g. chronic pulmonary disease, cardiovascular disease), which may influence the patient's fitness for surgery.

One good example of the relevance of the features of pain in reading a diagnosis is acute appendicitis – a condition likely to be discussed rather than seen in surgical finals.

The typical history of appendicitis is of progressive onset of colicky central abdominal pain (Fig. 6.15a). This moves to become a localized pain in the right iliac fossa (Fig. 6.15b) over McBurney's point (a point

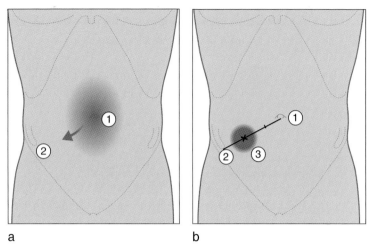

a   b

Fig. 6.15 In appendicitis, progressive onset of colicky central abdominal pain: (a) moving to become a localized pain in the right iliac fossa and (b) deep to McBurney's point.

① Umbilicus   ② Anterosuperior iliac spine   ③ x = McBurney's point

two-thirds along a line between the umbilicus and the anterosuperior iliac spine) as the peritoneum of the abdominal wall becomes involved in the inflammatory process. Associated features may include anorexia; initially, there may be vomiting and a loose bowel motion. As a result of the extensive differential diagnosis (Fig. 6.16), ask about a recent upper respiratory tract infection (which may be associated with mesenteric adenitis) and urinary symptoms (which may also occur in appendicitis with irritation of the bladder by the appendix), and in females aged 10–60 take a careful menstrual history.

Beware, as pain perceived to be in the abdomen may be referred to the upper abdomen from organs superior to the diaphragm, particularly the heart (e.g. with angina or myocardial infarction) or the lung and pleurae (e.g. in pneumonia, lung infarction). In the case of women, do not forget the gynaecological causes of abdominal pain, including pelvic inflammatory disease, endometriosis and ovarian cyst rupture. Rare conditions (at least in surgical finals) that may present with abdominal pain include coeliac disease and irritable bowel syndrome (shortened to IBS, causing potential confusion with inflammatory bowel disease if you are not careful). IBS does, however, affect up to 25% of the general population.

Fig. 6.16 Differential diagnosis of appendicitis.

1 Mesenteric adenitis
2 Meckel's diverticulitis
3 Terminal ileum inflammatory bowel disease
4 Caecal cancer
5 Inflamed fallopian tube/fimbria
6 Ovarian cyst – or torted ovary

7 Ectopic pregnancy
8 Bladder infection
⑨ Uterus
⑩ Ileum
⑪ Ascending colon

EXAMINATION

Inspection, palpation, percussion and auscultation of the gastrointestinal system are required. These include examination of the hands, head and neck, mouth and abdomen. In addition you may need to examine the cardiorespiratory system if you think that the pain is referred from superior to the diaphragm.

If the physical examination and investigations are unremarkable, psychological assessment may be worthwhile but impossible in an exam setting!

INVESTIGATIONS

Investigations should begin with the urine and faeces, for signs of disease processes. An FBC and biochemistry, an erect chest radiograph in the acute setting to look for pneumoperitoneum (Fig. 6.17), a plain abdominal radiograph (Fig. 6.18) and an ultrasound scan (particularly valuable for gallstones) complete the first-line investigations.

The symptoms and signs may point towards the upper gastrointestinal tract, suggesting upper gastrointestinal endoscopy (with biopsy for *Helicobacter pylori*) or barium studies, or to the lower gastrointestinal tract, suggesting colonoscopy or barium studies.

Coeliac disease is diagnosed after duodenal biopsy and the detection of anti-gliadin antibodies.

Renal colic*

HISTORY

Patients with renal colic make good subjects for surgical finals because they are usually under 65, give a concise history and may have clear radiographs.

A classic history of renal colic is the rapid onset of unilateral loin pain radiating into the groin (and in males to the testis) on the same side. The pain is usually caused by a small stone passing from the renal pelvis (Fig. 6.19) down the ureter, driven on by waves of ureteric peristalsis (hence the waves of colicky pain). The pain is usually sufficiently severe to elicit nausea and vomiting, pallor and sweating but, unlike many causes of acute abdominal pain, may be more bearable if the patient moves around. There may be a history of previous similar episodes, relieved by analgesia (NSAIDs are as effective as opiates).

Ask about a history of living or working in hot conditions, excess milk ingestion or a family history of stone disease. Urinary tract stones may be associated with urinary tract infections or known anatomical variants.

KEY POINTS

- Renal colic can be diagnosed on the typical history
- Microscopic haematuria can confirm the diagnosis
- Intravenous urography may demonstrate a stone

Fig. 6.17 Erect chest radiograph in a patient with a perforated peptic ulcer.

1 Free intraperitoneal air   ② Diaphragm   ③ Liver

EXAMINATION

On inspection, the patient my be pale, sweating and restless and, if there is also urinary tract infection, pyrexial. Palpation of the abdomen may identify renal angle tenderness, tenderness in the iliac fossa of the affected side but no rebound or guarding. Percussion and auscultation are not usually helpful.

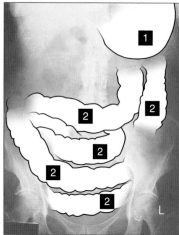

Fig. 6.18 Plain radiograph of small bowel obstruction.

1 Distended stomach   **2** Distended small bowel loops

Fig. 6.19 Normal anatomy of urinary system.

① Right kidney   ② Left kidney   ③ Renal pelvis   ④ Ureter   ⑤ Bladder

INVESTIGATION

Urinary testing and microscopy will demonstrate microscopic haematuria and protein, and may show crystals. Blood testing shows a raised WCC, though usually biochemistry is normal. Plain abdominal radiology may let you identify a stone in the line of the ureter or additional stones in the renal pelvis or bladder. Intravenous urography (Fig. 6.20) of intravenous contrast excreted by the kidneys very effectively outlines the upper urinary tract and may delineate a stone obstructing the ureter.

MANAGEMENT

Most stones pass from the ureter unaided into the bladder and so analgesia is the main treatment. Some stones lodge, usually as the ureter passes through the bladder wall, and require lithotriptic destruction or endoscopic removal.

Fig. 6.20 Intravenous urogram.

1 Dilated renal pelvis   ④ Normal urinary tract
2 Dilated ureter   ⑤ Bladder
3 Stone

Inflammatory bowel disease*

HISTORY

Patients with inflammatory bowel disease (Crohn's disease, ulcerative colitis) often have a complex history, and many have had multiple hospital admissions and may have had several surgical operations. Fortunately, most patients are well versed in the chronology of their disease, the management of complications (such as obstruction, fistulae, stomas), the medications that they are on or have taken in the past and dietary changes or supplements. Complexity can make for a rambling history. When you present the patient to your examiners, make sure that you have the key events clear: diagnosis and how it was made; attempts at medical treatment; and surgical procedures – what was done, when and why. State how the disease has affected that individual – not only the symptoms of pain, diarrhoea, etc. but also whether it has meant giving up work, missing time from college or university, significantly curtailing social activities.

Questions about gastrointestinal symptoms should obtain information about mouth ulcers, dysphagia, abdominal pain (upper, central or lower abdominal pain, which may or may not be well localized), nausea, vomiting, diarrhoea (with blood or mucus), constipation, abdominal masses, jaundice/itch (related to hepatobiliary disease), fistulae to the abdominal wall, perianal abscesses and anal fistulae. Other (systemic) manifestations relate to eye symptoms, skin rashes (erythema nodosum or pyoderma gangrenosum), arthropathies and weight loss.

There may be a family history of inflammatory bowel disease.

KEY POINTS

- Inflammatory bowel disease may affect multiple systems
- Remember that the patient is an individual. How do the symptoms affect the patient?

EXAMINATION

On inspection, look for signs of malnutrition or anaemia (caused by blood loss or vitamin B_{12} malabsorption as a result of terminal ileum malfunction or resection) and for signs of skin disease (e.g. erythema nodosum). Crohn's disease, in particular, can give rise to signs from the lips at one end to the perianal skin at the other, so you will need to examine both ends of the gastrointestinal tract, and all that lies between, where you can.

Abdominal examination may be complicated by the presence of a scar or stoma (and sometimes more than one of each). The patient will often know exactly what type of stoma it is and allow you to confirm the presence of a spout (indicating an ileostomy). Multiple scars (which may be in unusual sites, and sometimes quite distorted as a result of postoperative sepsis) and fistulae (communications between two surfaces lined by epithelium) can also make abdominal examination difficult. Anal fistulae, usually after perianal abscess formation, can be a feature of Crohn's disease. The fistula may be simple (Figs 6.21 and 6.22) or complex, even requiring an ileostomy to relieve symptoms. It can be

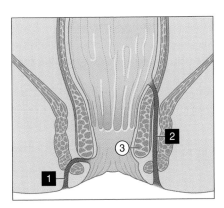

Fig. 6.21 Anatomy of anorectal fistulae.

1 Superficial fistula
2 High fistula
③ Internal sphincter

Fig. 6.22 Fistula.

1 Superficial fistula
② Anus
③ Anal orifice

helpful, in a long case, to make a sketch of what you see and find, to refer to or to show to the examiners.

INVESTIGATION

A basic FBC (to detect anaemia, which may be microcytic as a result of iron deficiency, or macrocytic) and blood biochemistry should be obtained, including LFTs to detect biliary involvement. Trace element measurement (e.g. zinc, selenium) may be required if the patient is chronically malnourished. Markers of inflammation, including ESR and CRP, may be useful as indicators of disease activity.

Radiological investigations should include plain abdominal films (in the acute situation for loops of bowel, toxic dilatation of the colon or bowel obstruction). Contrast studies can provide useful information. A small-bowel enema (the patient swallows a nasoenteric tube, down which contrast is injected) or small-bowel follow-through (after the patient has had a drink of contrast) can be used to examine the small intestine for strictures and fistulae. A barium enema can provide useful information about colonic strictures (Fig. 6.23), mucosal abnormalities or fistulae to other parts of the bowel or bladder.

Fig. 6.23 Contrast enema showing Crohn's disease of the colon with stricture formation.

1 Colonic strictures   **4** Rectum
2 Transverse colon   **5** Radio-opaque gallstones (incidental finding)
3 Descending colon

Endoscopic examination may include upper gastrointestinal endoscopy, small bowel enteroscopy (if available) and colonoscopy. Colonoscopic screening of patients with long-standing ulcerative colitis should be considered because of the cancer risk. Patients with perianal Crohn's disease are particularly prone to fistulae and abscess formation, and so may require an examination under anaesthesia for adequate assessment of anorectal disease.

There is great overlap between ulcerative colitis and Crohn's disease, so we have lumped them together but examiners will often ask about the differences between these two conditions. Table 6.3 will remind you of some of the key differences.

Pancreatitis*

Pancreatitis can be classified as acute, recurrent/relapsing or chronic. Of acute cases 80% will resolve spontaneously without problems, but the 20% of patients who develop severe pancreatitis or complications are often seriously ill. A minority of patients will develop chronic pancreatitis, and others will have recurrent attacks of acute pancreatitis, being well between exacerbations. Recurrent attacks may occur because the agent responsible for the pancreatitis (e.g. alcohol) persists. Table 6.4 lists the causes of pancreatitis. If you have a patient with pancreatitis in surgical finals you should endeavour to:

Table 6.3 Key differences between ulcerative colitis and Crohn's disease		
	Ulcerative colitis	**Crohn's disease**
Age group	Generally 18–40 years	Bimodal 18–30+ >65 years
Site	Incontinuity proximally from the rectum	Skip lesions affecting any part of the gastrointestinal tract Classically terminal ileum
Presentation	Per rectal bleeding and diarrhoea	Dependent on site
Radiology	Loss of haustral pattern and shallow ulcers on barium enema	Rose-thorn ulcers on barium enema Strictures and fistulae
	Plain films may show acute dilatation in emergency presentation	Distribution as above

Table 6.4 Causes of pancreatitis

Frequency of occurrence	Cause
Common (80% of cases in the UK)	Gallstones Alcohol
Intermediate	Trauma (post-ERCP, blunt abdominal trauma) Tumour (ampullary or pancreatic) Drugs (e.g. azathioprine, β blockers, steroids) Infection (e.g. viruses, particularly mumps) Hyperlipidaemia Hypothermia
Rare	Metabolic (e.g. hypercalcaemia) Congenital (e.g. pancreas divisum)
10% of cases	Idiopathic
Mention scorpion sting to your examiners at your peril!	

- find the aetiological agent
- define the pattern of the patient's disease
- assess the severity of the attack.

The cause of the pancreatitis, and whether the patient is recovering from acute pancreatitis or has chronic pancreatitis, may be evident from the history. The most life-threatening complications of acute pancreatitis include renal failure, respiratory failure and cardiac failure, in addition to the necrosis (with or without supervening haemorrhage or sepsis) that may occur in the pancreatic bed. Malnutrition and narcotic (opiate) dependence are common complications of chronic pancreatitis.

KEY POINTS

- Acute pancreatitis is usually secondary to gallstones or alcohol
- Diagnosis by elevated amylase (>3 × normal)
- There are prognostic criteria for the severity of acute pancreatitis
- Treatment is largely supportive

HISTORY

Ask about pain, which is classically epigastric, radiating to the back and, in the acute situation, alleviated by leaning forwards or pacing around.

In acute pancreatitis, the pain and rigid abdomen may mimic a perforated viscus. The pain may be exacerbated by precipitating factors (particularly alcohol), associated with nausea and vomiting and only relieved by strong (opiate) analgesia. Record the number of painful episodes, and find out whether the pain resolves completely between attacks.

In the case of chronic pancreatitis, particular questions should be asked about malabsorption (weight loss, stool difficult to flush away and offensive), diabetes (usually type 1), analgesic use, previous investigations (such as ultrasonography, ERCP and CT) and previous surgery.

It is important to try to determine the cause of the pancreatitis (usually gallstones or alcohol), and so questions must be asked about previous and current alcohol intake. A history of biliary colic, with or without jaundice and with or without fever, may suggest that gallstones are the underlying cause. The patient's occupation should be noted, particularly if it gives easy access to alcohol.

EXAMINATION

With the patient adequately exposed, look for signs of jaundice, bruising, or malnutrition (caused by alcohol abuse, pancreatic insufficiency or chronic liver disease). Some of these signs may be evident on examination of the hands and torso, but examination of the abdomen will yield much more information. Inspection of the abdomen may reveal an abdominal mass (e.g. a pseudocyst or carcinoma). There may be scars from previous biliary or pancreatic surgery, but there will obviously be no evidence of ERCP. There may be drains, to drain either the pancreatic bed or a pleural effusion secondary to the pancreatic inflammation. There may be a feeding tube passing into the jejunum, or a gastrostomy drainage tube to the stomach. Look for bruising (although neither the classic Cullen's periumbilical bruising nor the Grey–Turner flank bruising of acute pancreatitis are likely to be present in a patient used for exams). There may be signs of portal hypertension (e.g. caput medusae).

Ask whether the abdomen is tender or sore, and if so be particularly gentle when examining these areas. Palpate for hepatomegaly, splenomegaly, a pancreatic pseudocyst and pancreatic carcinoma, either of the last two usually being palpable as a central abdominal mass. It is worth listening for a succussion splash, in case there is gastric outflow obstruction.

Percussion may confirm a mass, but auscultation with a stethoscope in surgical finals is unlikely to be useful in the abdominal examination.

However, auscultation of the chest may demonstrate the side(s), size and extent of a unilateral or bilateral pleural effusion and the associated pulmonary features, particularly in a patient recovering from acute pancreatitis.

INVESTIGATIONS

The aims of the investigations are to establish the diagnosis of pancreatitis, assess its severity and suggest the appropriate therapy. The diagnosis and early prognostic criteria in acute pancreatitis may be based on: testing blood and urine for hyperamylasaemia (3 × the upper limit of normal − useful in diagnosis only); high blood glucose level; renal impairment; abnormal LFTs; poor arterial blood oxygenation; a raised WCC; anaemia; and abnormal coagulation (Table 6.5). Beware that ischaemic bowel, acute cholecystitis or a perforated duodenal ulcer can also lead to hyperamylasaemia.

Useful information may be obtained from a chest radiograph (particularly in the case of pleural effusions) or from ultrasonography (for gallstones in particular, although the pancreas and any pseudocyst may be visualized). A plain abdominal film may demonstrate gas/fluid levels associated with ileus caused by the pancreatitis. Also useful in appropriate circumstances is CT (with contrast enhancement − Fig. 6.24) to assess the swelling and necrosis of an acutely inflamed pancreas or to

Table 6.5 Early prognostic criteria for severity of acute pancreatitis

Criterion	Threshold
Age of patient	>55 years
White blood cells	$>15 \times 10^9/l$
Glucose (in blood)	>10 mmol/l
Urea	>16 mmol/l
PaO_2	<8 kPa
Calcium	<2.0 mmol/l
Albumin	<32 g/l
LDH (lactate dehydrogenase)	>600 IU/l
ALT (alanine aminotransferase)	>100 U/l

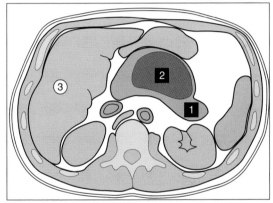

Fig. 6.24 CT scan in acute pancreatitis.

1 Inflamed pancreas   **2** Pancreatic pseudocyst   ③ Liver

visualize one or more pseudocysts, an atrophic pancreas or a pancreatic carcinoma. Portal hypertension, in chronic alcoholic pancreatitis associated with alcoholic liver disease, may also be apparent from a CT scan. ERCP with sphincterotomy, to remove a stone obstructing the ampulla of Vater or to assess the anatomy of the pancreatic duct in chronic pancreatitis, may also be useful.

Pancreatic exocrine insufficiency may be suggested by offensive, putty-like, yellow stool, and can be confirmed by measuring faecal fat content (with the patient on a suitable diet) or by the pancreatolauryl test (for pancreatic esterase activity). Pancreatic endocrine function can be assessed by a glucose tolerance test, if the patient is not overtly diabetic.

MANAGEMENT

The treatment of acute pancreatitis is conservative unless there are specific complications. Treatment should be as follows: analgesics (many prefer pethidine, which is said to cause least spasm of the sphincter of Oddi); fluid replacement (patients should be fasted and will require maintenance intravenous fluids, but in addition may have large nasogastric aspirates and peritoneal exudates); and monitoring, to ensure that complications are detected and treated promptly. Patients with severe disease warrant high-dependency type care. Patients may need physiotherapy because of pain and bed rest. Some will develop ARDS (acute respiratory distress syndrome) and will need ventilatory support.

Patients with severe pancreatitis who do not improve rapidly should be considered for ERCP and sphincterotomy if common bile duct stones are confirmed. A minority of patients will develop a pancreatic abscess or a pseudocyst, in which case percutaneous or surgical drainage of necrotic/infected material or a mature cyst may be needed.

The long-term care of patients with acute pancreatitis should be aimed at preventing further attacks. This may involve a cholecystectomy if gallstones have been implicated as the causative agent, or it may involve emphatic advice about drinking habits or altering medications.

The management of chronic pancreatitis is a more long-term problem. Obviously every attempt should be made to remove aetiological factors. In addition, patients may need analgesics, insulin replacement and pancreatic extracts on a long-term basis. Surgery may be required for patients with intractable pain, and may involve either decompression of an obstructed pancreatic duct or resection of the pancreas. The latter will, however, condemn the patient to long-term insulin and pancreatic extract replacement therapy.

Rectal bleeding*

For the purposes of surgical finals, rectal bleeding is most commonly the result of haemorrhoids, carcinoma, polyps, diverticular disease, inflammatory bowel disease or angiodysplasia.

KEY POINTS

- The history will suggest the likely diagnosis
- Investigation of rectal bleeding aims to exclude life-threatening conditions

HISTORY

The key questions about rectal bleeding concern the colour of the blood and when the blood is seen. In general, bright red blood is rectal/anal in origin, dark blood is colonic and melaena signals blood from the proximal gastrointestinal tract. Fresh red blood on toilet paper only is likely to be from haemorrhoids; red blood on the stool is likely to be from a rectal lesion; and red or dark blood mixed in with the stool is likely to be from a colonic lesion. Bleeding due to diverticular disease may be sudden and profuse, but may stop spontaneously.

Haemorrhoids

These remain poorly understood but it is helpful to know a classification for communication with colleagues. First-degree haemorrhoids are not visible on inspection of the anus, or palpable on digital rectal examination, but can be seen on proctoscopy. Second-degree haemorrhoids prolapse through the anal margin but spontaneously return into the anal canal. Third-degree haemorrhoids have prolapsed but will return into the anal canal with manipulation. A fourth-degree haemorrhoid cannot be replaced into the anal canal and may be thrombosed. Haemorrhoids originating from the anorectal mucosa are sometimes known as internal haemorrhoids or piles (Fig. 6.25), and a perianal haematoma at the anal–skin margin is confusingly known as a thrombosed external pile.

There is typically a history of constipation, anal discomfort (rather than pain), red spotting of blood on toilet paper and mucus staining of underwear. There may be episodes of prolapse of the haemorrhoids, spontaneously returning, requiring manual replacement. Most patients

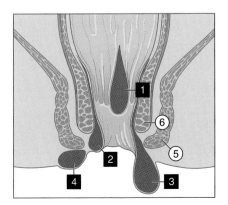

Fig. 6.25 Anatomy of haemorrhoids.

1 First-degree haemorrhoid
2 Second-degree haemorrhoid
3 Third-degree haemorrhoid
4 Perianal haematoma ('external pile')
5 External sphincter
6 Internal sphincter

Fig. 6.26 Anal fissure and haemorrhoid.

1 Fissure
2 Sentinel tags
3 Internal sphincter
4 Haemorrhoid
⑤ Anal orifice

know the diagnosis, but concomitant colorectal or anal neoplasia must be excluded.

A previous history of dull LIF pain in a patient who has rectal bleeding may indicate diverticular disease. The colicky pain of bowel obstruction associated with blood in the stool may be the result of a carcinoma. Pain on defecation is a classic symptom of an anal fissure (Fig. 6.26), which may result in a small amount of fresh blood on the stool and toilet paper. There may be mucus production (e.g. from a rectal adenoma) or blood/faecal staining of underwear (from haemorrhoids). Important symptoms that may be associated with bleeding are a change in bowel habit, or the recent onset of constipation or diarrhoea, any of which may occur with colorectal cancer or diverticular disease.

Ask about complications, e.g. colovesical fistula, which may present as recurrent urinary tract infections, dirty-coloured urine or (rarely) classic pneumaturia. Also ask about septic episodes and hospital admissions. A history of surgery for a polyp (usually performed via a colonoscope), for a cancer or previously for haemorrhoids or a fissure is worth noting.

A family history of colorectal cancer, polyps or inflammatory bowel disease is also important.

EXAMINATION

While taking a history, you may be able to assess whether a patient shows outward signs of systemic disease, such as cachexia.

Abdominal examination, of an appropriately positioned and exposed patient, should follow the scheme already outlined, with particular attention paid on inspection to scars, stomas and visible masses.

A diverticular mass or a tumour mass may be palpable. The colon, containing faeces, may be palpable proximal to a segment of diverticular disease or a colonic neoplasm. Remember to palpate for the liver, particularly if you suspect a colonic cancer.

Percussion should be used to confirm the resonance or dullness of any mass that you can palpate, and to help delineate the position of the liver.

INVESTIGATIONS

Dipstick testing of the urine may detect blood and protein. If there is a colovesical fistula, urine cultures grow gut organisms.

An FBC may detect a microcytic anaemia if there is sufficient chronic blood loss. If there is ongoing inflammation, the WCC may be raised.

However, the key investigations are endoscopic examination of the anal canal (proctoscopy), rectum (sigmoidoscopy) and colon (colonoscopy – Fig. 6.27) or barium enema, followed by ultrasonography of the abdomen (supplemented by CT) to detect liver metastases or inflammatory masses.

Colorectal cancer*

Colorectal cancer is common both in real life and in surgical finals. The presenting complaints can be non-specific (including rectal bleeding –

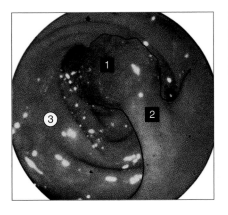

Fig. 6.27 Polyp in colon.

1 Bleeding polyp
2 Stalk
③ Normal colon

see above) and may cause diagnostic confusion with diverticular disease, IBS or haemorrhoids.

HISTORY

When taking a history, ask about vague lower abdominal discomfort and bloatedness, which are common. The classic symptoms are fresh bleeding on or mixed with the stool (for rectal/sigmoid carcinoma), change in bowel habit (constipation or loose, frequent stools), or symptoms of anaemia (breathlessness, tiredness) secondary to blood loss from right-sided colon or caecal cancer. Rectal cancers (and adenomas) may produce considerable mucus. Rectal cancers may also give a feeling of urgency (tenesmus) or incomplete emptying and, if locally advanced, may cause perineal pain or involve the sphincters to result in faecal incontinence.

A family history of colon cancer (particularly first-degree relatives under the age of 45), polyposis or a past history of polyps, ulcerative colitis or Crohn's disease increases the risk of developing colorectal cancer. A second (metachronous) carcinoma occurs in some 5% of individuals, so ask about any previous history of colorectal cancer.

The patient may have been taking medication to relieve constipation and iron (causing black stools) to improve anaemia.

EXAMINATION

Look for general signs of gastrointestinal disease or malignancy. Weight loss, jaundice (secondary to liver metastases) and debility are late signs of advanced disease. Pallor or leukonychia secondary to anaemia may be evident.

On inspection of the abdomen, there may be no outward sign of the carcinoma within. In thin individuals with a large lesion, a mass may be visible, or the backlog of faeces behind a progressively obstructing colonic carcinoma may be evident as a mass. An obstructing carcinoma may present signs of large bowel obstruction. A grossly enlarged liver secondary to liver metastases may be visible in a cachectic individual.

On palpation, gentle palpation followed by deeper palpation of the abdomen may delineate a palpable colonic mass; it should be possible to indent a faecal mass, whereas a palpable cancer is solid but may be mobile (given the mesentery, for example, of the sigmoid colon). The size, position and fixity of the mass can be described.

Rectal (per anal) examination is crucial to identifying the presence of a lesion in the rectum. If a lump or mass is palpable, it is important to describe its position (anterior, posterior, lateral), distance from the anorectal junction (which may dictate whether the anus can be preserved during surgery for a cancer), size/extent, mobility (e.g. highly mobile like a polyp – see Fig. 6.27) or fixity (e.g. a rectal carcinoma invading the sacral tissues), and the involvement of other structures (such as the vagina). If the rectal mucosa feels normal, a sample of stool, if present, can be removed on the gloved digit to test for faecal occult blood, which may be the only indication on clinical examination of a polyp or carcinoma lurking proximally in the colon.

Percussion can be used to assess whether an abdominal mass is apparently more solid than the surrounding tympanic normal bowel. Percussion for shifting dullness can also be used to look for ascites. Auscultation may be normal in a patient with colorectal carcinoma, although, if the cancer obstructs the bowel, sounds may become obstructive.

INVESTIGATIONS

An FBC should look for microcytic anaemia from blood loss into the colon. Plasma viscosity/ESR may be raised. Urea and creatinine may be elevated in advanced cancer of the rectum (resulting from ureteric obstruction) and abnormal LFTs may signify liver metastases. A grossly raised CEA may also suggest the presence of metastases.

A plain radiograph of the chest and an ultrasound scan of the liver should be used to seek metastatic disease. A contrast-enhanced CT scan or MR scan may be used to look for liver metastases and assess local invasion by a rectal cancer. For patients admitted with large bowel (colonic) obstruction secondary to a colon cancer (Fig. 6.28), plain abdominal radiographs can demonstrate the obstruction (Fig. 6.29).

Before surgery on the colon or rectum, all of the large bowel needs to be imaged for synchronous second cancers or polyps (see Fig. 6.27). In the clinic, rigid sigmoidoscopy and proctoscopy can supplement rectal examination to visualize, to assess invasion using endoscopic ultrasonography and to biopsy a rectal cancer. Barium enema examination (single contrast, see Fig. 6.30, or double contrast using contrast plus air) can outline the remaining colon to the terminal ileum, provided that the bowel is adequately cleared first (usually using oral purgative solutions), although colonoscopy in experienced hands may have the advantage of allowing biopsy of any visible abnormalities. In some centres, a combination of barium enema and flexible sigmoidoscopy is used to ensure that the sigmoid colon (which has a high incidence of

Fig. 6.28 Colon carcinoma.

1 Colon cancer
② Normal colon

Fig. 6.29 Erect abdominal radiograph in large bowel obstruction.

1 Distended proximal bowel
2 Loops of small bowel with thickened wall
3 Gas/fluid levels in colon
4 Gas/fluid levels in small bowel

5 Nasogastric tube
⑥ Transverse colon
⑦ Liver

Fig. 6.30 Single-contrast barium enema of rectosigmoid cancer.

1 Apple-core deformity, rectosigmoid junction   ③ Rectum
② Sigmoid colon   **4** Tube to instil contrast

cancers – see Fig. 6.30 – and is more difficult to visualize on barium enema) is adequately examined.

TREATMENT

The mainstay of treatment is surgical resection of the cancer (see Fig. 6.28) together with the draining lymph nodes, and is based on the anatomical blood supply of the colon (Fig. 6.31) such that any anastomosis has the greatest chance of healing. For rectal cancers, mesorectal excision of the tissues around the rectum is required to get clearance around the cancer. Under circumstances where an anastomosis is ill advised (emergency surgery) or impossible (an abdominoperineal resection of the rectum), a colostomy (see Fig. 6.5) or ileostomy will be necessary. On the basis of Dukes' staging (Table 6.6) and TNM (tumour, nodes, metastases) staging, further adjuvant therapy may be given. Postoperative chemotherapy for Dukes' C cancers and preoperative or postoperative radiotherapy for rectal cancer can be used as additional therapy to reduce the chances of systemic and local disease recurrence respectively.

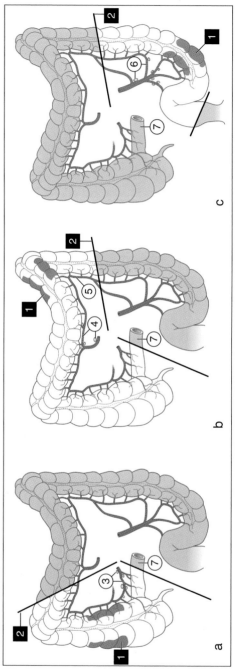

Fig. 6.31 Surgical resection: (a) right hemicolectomy, (b) extended right hemicolectomy, (c) anterior resection. Healthy (pink) bowel can be anastomosed after resection of the cancer.

1 Cancer	3 Ileocolic artery and nodes	5 Marginal artery	7 Ileum
2 Extent of resection	4 Middle colic artery and nodes	6 Inferior mesenteric artery and nodes	

Diverticular disease*

Diverticular disease (see Fig. 6.32), similar to colorectal cancer, is increasingly common with age and so patients are also found with diverticular disease in surgical finals. Inflammation of one or more diverticula, a process known as diverticulitis (Fig 6.33) may cause marked symptoms, although many people with uncomplicated diverticular disease are asymptomatic. The presenting complaints can be non-specific and may cause diagnostic confusion with colorectal cancer, inflammatory bowel disease or IBS.

HISTORY

In the history, ask about lower abdominal discomfort and bloatedness, which are common. Constipation, pelleted stools, offensive flatus, mucus from the anus and blood mixed in with the stool are symptoms strongly associated with diverticular disease. On occasion, diverticular disease may present with a brisk fresh rectal bleed (Fig. 6.33) from the neck of a diverticulum, which is alarming to the patient but usually self-limiting. These are also classic symptoms of colorectal cancer and both conditions may occur in the same individual, hence, even in the presence of known diverticular disease, any new symptoms should be

Fig. 6.32 Double-contrast enema demonstrating diverticular disease (radiographs taken with the patient lying on his side).

1 Diverticula	③ Transverse colon	⑤ Rectum
2 Contrast level	④ Sigmoid colon	⑥ Rectal catheter

Table 6.6 Dukes' classification

Dukes' A	Cancer confined to colon wall
Dukes' B	Cancer penetrating colon wall
Dukes' C_1	Involving mesenteric lymph nodes
Dukes' C_2	Most proximal node (in resection specimen) involved with tumour
Dukes' D	Distant (liver) metastases[a]

[a]Dukes' D is used clinically but was not originally described by Cuthbert Dukes.

Fig. 6.33 Complications of diverticular disease.

1 Perforation
2 Gas, faeces, etc. from perforation
3 Acute inflammation
4 Thick wall, narrow lumen stricture
5 Bleeding
6 Fistula – to bladder (bladder not shown)

7 Abscess
8 Descending colon
9 Sigmoid colon
10 Rectum
11 Transverse colon

investigated to exclude the recent development of a colorectal cancer. Fistulation from a diverticulum to the bladder (resulting in symptoms of frequent urinary tract infection as a result of gut organisms that recurs despite adequate antibiotic treatment, or even pneumaturia), to another part of the bowel, to the vagina (particularly in a woman who has had a hysterectomy, resulting in a brown offensive vaginal discharge) may cause symptoms. Local abscess formation may result in complaints of localized tenderness and fever.

The patient may have been taking medication to relieve the constipation caused by the thickened walls and narrowed lumen of a colon affected by diverticular disease.

EXAMINATION

On examination, there may be signs of systemic upset (fever) or blood loss (pallor) as a result of complications of diverticular disease. However, most patients show few systemic signs on presentation.

On inspection of the abdomen, a diverticular mass may be visible in the LIF, secondary to local inflammation or abscess formation. On palpation, gentle superficial then deep palpation of the abdomen may delineate a palpable sigmoid colon, the bowel most frequently involved in diverticular disease. On rectal examination, a tender diverticular mass may be palpable on the left side, although the rectal wall should feel normal. A stool specimen should be tested for faecal occult blood. Vaginal examination with a speculum will be appropriate if there is a history of vaginal discharge suggestive of a fistula.

Percussion can be used to assess whether an abdominal mass is solid relative to the surrounding tympanic normal bowel. After perforation (Fig. 6.33) large amounts of free peritoneal air may make the abdomen tympanic. Auscultation should be normal unless the diverticular disease causes bowel obstruction (Fig. 6.33) or peritonitis secondary to perforation.

INVESTIGATION

Urine testing should be used to look for evidence of urinary infection from a diverticular fistula.

Blood tests include an FBC and measurement of plasma viscosity, looking for microcytic anaemia from blood loss into the colon and a raised WCC and plasma viscosity secondary to inflammation. Plain abdominal and erect chest films may demonstrate free intraperitoneal air. An ultrasound, CT or MR scan of the abdomen may demonstrate a diverticular mass. In the absence of acute symptoms, rigid or flexible sigmoidoscopy combined with contrast enema examination (usually double contrast with barium plus air – see Fig. 6.32) can outline the diseased bowel and ensure that the sigmoid colon is adequately visualized.

MANAGEMENT

Symptom control using dietary manipulation and antispasmodics, antibiotics for episodes of inflammation and careful observation and intravenous support at the time of acute, self-limiting bleeding mean that colonic resection is required only for complications of diverticular disease (see Fig. 6.33): perforation, obstruction, fistulation, abscess formation and major haemorrhage.

Abdominal aortic aneurysm**

Most aneurysms are degenerative in origin and associated with atherosclerotic disease elsewhere in the cardiovascular system. Inflammatory aneurysms are comparatively rare (if you touch on this topic in your exam, immunological tests for syphilis may be mentioned).

KEY POINT

- Back/loin pain mimicking renal colic ± a hypotensive episode in an elderly patient is suggestive of a leaking abdominal aortic aneurysm

---

HISTORY

An abdominal aortic aneurysm (AAA) may be asymptomatic or cause back pain. A leaking aneurysm may present with back pain or loin pain, a history of collapse or a hypotensive episode in the acute context (beware when examining an elderly patient who has collapsed with 'renal colic' – he or she may well have a leaking AAA). If you have the opportunity (e.g. in a long case), ask whether the patient has any other history of peripheral, cardiac or cerebral vascular disease, and whether he or she smokes.

EXAMINATION

Remember to seek features of peripheral vascular disease on inspection (e.g. skin changes, ulceration, ischaemia, gangrene, amputation), palpation (pulses) and auscultation (bruits).

On abdominal examination, an aortic aneurysm (Fig. 6.34) is a mass that is expansile, centrally positioned (although it may be more prominent on the left- or right-hand side) and sometimes tender. Normal aortic pulsation may be visible on inspection, and may be readily palpable in a thin, normal person. In an elderly person the aorta may be ectatic, and it may be difficult to be sure that it is not aneurysmal.

Palpate the aorta using two digits, as described earlier, to delineate the extent of the expansile abdominal mass.

Auscultate for a bruit over the aorta, iliac vessels and renal arteries.

INVESTIGATION

A plain radiograph/lateral film (see Fig. 6.34) or CT scan (Fig. 6.35) of the abdomen may show the calcified wall of the aneurysm. However, an ultrasound scan should allow accurate measurement of the size and extent of the aneurysm, including any extension into the iliac vessels or proximal to the renal vessels. Increasing size, particularly over 5 cm, leads to a greater chance of leakage from or rupture of the aneurysm.

Fig. 6.34 Plain radiograph of abdominal aortic aneurysm.

1 Calcified wall of aneurysm	③ Lumbar vertebra
② Psoas muscle shadow	④ Site of enlarging umbilicus = ×

Fig. 6.35 CT scan of abdominal aortic aneurysm.

1 Aneurysm of aorta
② Lumbar vertebra
③ Psoas muscle

Splenomegaly**

Splenomegaly may be caused by: portal hypertension/occlusion; haematological causes, e.g. lymphoma (causing fever, weight loss and lymph node enlargement), leukaemia (particularly CLL [chronic lymphocytic leukaemia]), myelofibrosis, Felty syndrome (with rheumatoid arthritis) or infective causes (particularly Epstein–Barr virus and malaria). Occasionally, patients with a large spleen turn up in the exam – the most likely causes of splenomegaly in this situation are CLL, myelofibrosis and infection.

HISTORY

Remember to ask about family history, travel abroad and infective contacts.

EXAMINATION

Distinguishing between the spleen and the left kidney may depend on the presence of a splenic notch, a dull percussion note overlying the mass, and the position of the spleen close to the costal margin (you cannot 'get above' the spleen, i.e. insert your fingers between the spleen and the costal margin). Both the spleen and the kidney move on inspiration, but the spleen may appear to move inferomedially and the kidney inferiorly only.

In most surgical splenomegaly cases, the spleen is just palpable.

INVESTIGATIONS

The key investigations are haematological (including blood films) and ultrasonography.

SUMMARY

There are some diagnoses and problems that come up with regularity in surgical finals. Table 6.7 lists the most common conditions, their typical features (not all of which have to be present in every patient) and one key investigation (although other investigations may also be helpful).

Table 6.7 Common abdominal cases

Condition	Typical features	Key diagnostic investigation
Biliary colic	Upper abdominal pain, increasing to plateau and dispersing after a few hours; may be described as a band around the upper (right) abdomen	Ultrasonography
Pancreatitis	*Acute:* severe epigastric pain, radiating to back; may imitate perforated ulcer	Serum/urine amylase
	Chronic: persistent abdominal/back pain, with exacerbations; features of pancreatic insufficiency	ERCP
Peptic ulcer	Dyspepsia; epigastric pain, worse or relieved on eating; patient wakens at night	Upper endoscopy
Renal colic	Severe right-/left-sided pain, radiating to the groin/testicle	Intravenous urogram
Colonic neoplasm	Rectal bleeding, anaemia, mucus, change in bowel habit	Colonoscopy
Diverticular disease	Left iliac fossa pain, pellet stools, diarrhoea/constipation, rectal bleeding	Barium enema
Bowel obstruction	Abdominal distension, colicky pain, vomiting	Plain radiograph

KEY QUESTIONS

1. What are causes of, and how would you investigate:
   - jaundice?
   - altered bowel habit?
   - rectal bleeding?
   - hepatomegaly?
   - ascites?
   - a mass in the right upper quadrant?
   - a mass in the left upper quadrant?
   - a mass in the RIF?
   - a mass in the LIF?
   - a central abdominal mass?
2. What problems might be encountered when operating on a jaundiced patient?
3. How would you assess a patient with dysphagia?
4. What are the differences between Crohn's disease and ulcerative colitis?
5. What are the features and complications of acute pancreatitis?

7

Hernias and the groin

A hernia is an abnormal protrusion of an organ or tissue from its normal body cavity or restraining sheath. In surgical finals (and postgraduate exams), hernias of the abdominal wall are very common short cases (particularly in the groin, in the midline or associated with incisions), because they are suitable for examination by several candidates. A patient in a long case may have a hiatus hernia along with other conditions.

Abdominal wall hernias generally are composed of a peritoneal sac, which passes through a defect in the abdominal wall – the neck (Fig 7.1a). The sac may be empty but when the patient strains a portion of the abdominal viscera may protrude into it (i.e. omentum, small bowel, large bowel or bladder). A small, tight hernial orifice may result in a hernia that is irreducible (Fig. 7.1b) (rather than reducible) and the contents may become obstructed (Fig. 7.1c) (e.g. the bowel) or strangulated (Fig. 7.1d) (e.g. fat, omentum or bowel). Strangulation (compromise of the blood supply to the contents of the hernial sac) results from venous occlusion, then arterial occlusion and consequent gangrene. Not surprisingly, morbidity and mortality follow. It follows from this discussion that not all hernias are reducible but reducibility is the cardinal sign that will distinguish a hernia from other abdominal or groin swellings.

A variation on this theme is a sliding hernia in which an organ forms part of the hernia sac (Fig. 7.2a). The danger in this situation is that the organ may be damaged during a surgical repair unless the situation is recognised. If only a part of the bowel wall is trapped within a hernia and strangulation occurs, this is known as Richter's hernia (Fig. 7.2b). You are unlikely to see such a case in an examination because this is a true surgical emergency; however, you may be asked about this complication.

There are two favourite kinds of hernia that come up in exams: the sliding hernia (Fig. 7.2a) and Richter's hernia (Fig. 7.2b). Even rarer hernias include Maydl's hernia (Fig. 7.2c), Littré's hernia (Fig. 7.2d) and

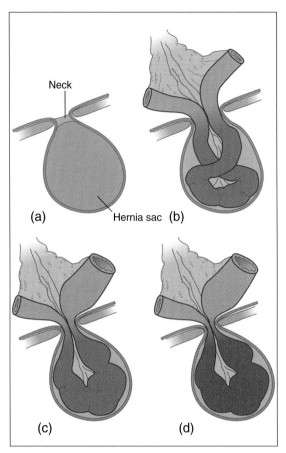

Fig. 7.1 (a) Hernia: the narrow point of a hernia where the hernial sac passes through the abdominal wall is known as the neck of the sac. This is usually the site of any strangulation. (b) Irreducible or incarcerated hernia: when the hernia contents cannot be returned to the abdominal cavity and the hernial sac cannot be reduced as a result of either adhesions of the contents of the sac or swelling of the tissues in the sac. (c) Obstructed hernia: when a loop of bowel within the hernia is obstructed. Note that the bowel leading into the hernia is dilated but the bowel leading from the hernia is collapsed. (d) Strangulated hernia: when the blood supply to the contents of a hernia is compromised. When a loop of gut is strangled, there will also be intestinal obstruction, then infarction and then perforation of the bowel.

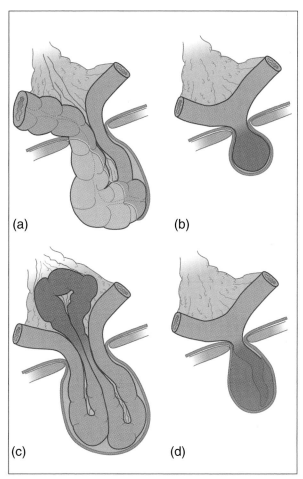

Fig. 7.2 (a) Sliding hernia: when tissues that are normally extraperitoneal, such as the bladder or colon, form part of the wall of the hernial sac. It is thought that the extraperitoneal tissue slides down the canal pulling the peritoneum with it. The sac can contain other loops of bowel, and the portion of gut that forms the hernia wall can become strangled. (b) Richter's hernia: part of the bowel wall is caught in the hernia. If the sac is small, a small section of bowel wall can be caught and strangled without causing intestinal obstruction. (c) Maydl's hernia: a rare variety of strangulation, when two loops of bowel are in the same sac. The intervening section of bowel in the abdomen is the first to suffer, and the strangulation is intra-abdominal. (d) Littré's hernia: strangulation of Meckel's diverticulum trapped in a hernial sac.

a pantaloon hernia (hernia to both sides of the inferior epigastric artery).

> ### KEY POINT
>
> - A small, tight, hernial orifice is more likely to entrap protuding organs than a wide neck to the hernia sac

TYPICAL CASES

Groin hernias*

The anatomy of the inguinal region is a favourite subject with examiners, and is well worth revising (Figs 7.3 and 7.4). Examiners also like to test you on the differences between indirect inguinal (Fig. 7.3), direct inguinal (Fig. 7.3) and femoral (Fig. 7.4) hernias: these may matter in clinical practice, because indirect inguinal hernias and (particularly) femoral hernias have a higher risk of strangulation compared with direct

Fig. 7.3 Bilateral inguinal hernia.

1a Indirect hernia sac	③ Femoral artery	⑥ Testis
1b Direct hernia sac	④ Inguinal ligament	⑦ Pubic tubercle
② Inferior epigastric artery	⑤ Spermatic cord	⑧ Deep inguinal ring

Fig. 7.4 Femoral hernia.

① Femoral hernia   ③ Inguinal ligament   ⑤ Femoral vein
② Femoral canal   ④ Femoral artery   ⑥ Pubic tubercle

hernias. However, it can sometimes be difficult to tell one from another, so a few hints are given in Table 7.1.

KEY POINTS

- Determine whether this is a femoral, direct inguinal or indirect inguinal hernia
- Is it reducible?
- Is it a recurrent hernia? (Look for a surgical scar)

HISTORY

The history of a groin swelling or a hernia should include the patient's age and occupation and a history of the swelling. Ask when the swelling first appeared, and whether it has changed in size or is tender. In the case of a hernia, is it reducible? Can it be pushed back (always, sometimes or only when lying down)? Does the patient have features that predispose to hernia formation:

- Respiratory (chronic cough)
- Gastrointestinal (constipation)
- Genitourinary (prostatism)

Table 7.1 Features of inguinal and femoral hernias

Features	Indirect inguinal hernia	Direct inguinal hernia	Femoral hernia
Typical patient	Younger male	Older male	Old female
Proportion of groin hernias (%)	60	25	15
Anatomy	Commences at deep ring, lateral to the inferior epigastric artery, and passes within the coverings of the spermatic cord	Bulges medial to the inferior epigastric artery	Emerges from the femoral canal
Relationship to the pubic tubercle	Starts lateral to and above the tubercle, but passes superomedial to the tubercle into the scrotum	Lies above the tubercle	Passes inferolateral to the tubercle
Descends into the scrotum?	Yes	No	No
Obstructs or strangulates?	Yes	Rarely	Yes

- Occupation (heavy lifting)
- Previous surgery
- Trauma
- Collagen diseases.

Is there only one hernia, or has the patient noticed another? Some patients have had previous hernia surgery, on the same side (so the hernia may be recurrent) or on the opposite side. They will know whether the hernia repair was performed as a child (when simple excision of the sac, herniotomy, will have been performed), or as an emergency or elective procedure. Until recently, hernia repair was performed by open surgery using sutures, but laparoscopic hernia repair and the use of prosthetic mesh have now become popular.

Ask about features that will influence fitness for anaesthesia and surgery, and the approach used:

- Cardiovascular disease
- Respiratory conditions
- Medications
- Allergies
- Past surgical history.

EXAMINATION

Examination should follow the standard routine of exposure/inspection, palpation, percussion and auscultation.

KEY POINTS

- Full exposure of the groin
- Examine the patient standing and lying down

It is traditional to examine the patient lying down first and then standing, because some small indirect or direct hernias are detectable only when a patient is standing. Remember to ask your examiner if you can examine the patient when standing. Full exposure of the groin area (including the scrotum in men) is needed to examine for hernias. Look first for surgical scars of open or laparoscopic hernia surgery: this can be more difficult than might be thought, because an old skin-crease incision can heal almost to invisibility, and may be camouflaged by pubic hair or folds of skin in obese patients. Visually identify any hernial orifices, and ask the patient to cough. Remember to look at both sides.

With the patient lying down, identify the palpable anatomical landmarks (Fig. 7.5):

- The pubic tubercle
- The anterosuperior iliac spine
- The femoral pulsation.

Now gently palpate the hernia and determine the following:

- Its position relative to the pubic tubercle (inguinal superior, femoral inferior)
- If it is reducible (many candidates try to reduce the hernia with the patient standing – this may be fruitless and will cause pain to the patient)

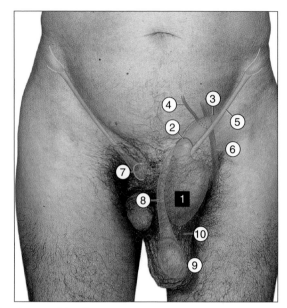

Fig. 7.5 Inguinoscrotal hernia.

1 Indirect hernia   ④ Inferior epigastric artery   ⑦ Pubic tubercle
② External ring   ⑤ Inguinal ligament   ⑧ Spermatic cord
③ Deep inguinal ring   ⑥ Femoral artery   ⑨ Testis
⑩ Site to examine to distinguish indirect hernia from testicular swelling
⑪ Anterosuperior iliac spine

- If it is an inguinal hernia, whether it is direct or indirect:
  - *direct* (see Fig. 7.3):
    - sac superior and lateral to pubic tubercle
    - not controlled by pressure over the internal ring
  - *indirect* (see Figs 7.3 and 7.5):
    - sac passes obliquely into scrotum, so is superior and medial to pubic tubercle; however, a large hernia may obscure the pubic tubercle
    - controlled by pressure over the deep inguinal ring (above the midpoint of the inguinal ligament; superolateral to the femoral pulse).
- If there is a contralateral hernia.

Percussion over a large hernia containing a hollow viscus (e.g. small bowel, colon) will be tympanic, whereas percussion of the omentum will not.

On auscultation over a hernia you may hear bowel sounds. You can comment on whether they sound normal (most likely in an exam) or obstructive (runs of high-pitched sounds), or are absent.

SUMMARY

If you are asked to summarise your findings after examining a groin hernia, you should certainly comment on the following:

- History:
  - age
  - length of time hernia has been present
  - has it changed?
  - initial precipitating factors
  - related factors, such as chronic cough
  - whether the hernia is painful and whether it reduces.
- Examination
  - position of hernia
  - type of hernia, i.e. inguinal (direct or indirect), femoral (and why you think it is)
  - reducible or not
  - likely contents if irreducible.

Other hernias

The locations of various types of abdominal wall hernia are shown in Fig, 7.6. All hernias should be gently manipulated to assess reducibility. Ask the patient whether the hernia can be reduced, and enlist his or her help if you are allowed. Identify the margins of the hernial orifice: strangulation is less likely in the case of a large defect than if the sac has a small, tight neck. If the hernia is reducible, try to control the neck of the sac and ask the patient to cough again.

Incisional hernias*

KEY POINTS

- Incisional hernias are often associated with previous wound complications (e.g. infection)
- A large diffuse hernia may be awkward to deal with but remember to determine whether or not it is reducible and to define the margins

Fig. 7.6 Location of hernias.

1 Epigastric
2 Divarication of the recti
3 Paraumbilical
4 Umbilical

5 Incisional
6 Previous hernia repair scar
7 Direct inguinal
8 Spigelian

9 Femoral
10 Indirect inguinal
⑪ Pubic tubercle
⑫ Inguinal ligament

HISTORY

Ask the patient about any previous operation(s), and any associated complications such as wound infection or dehiscence, which may have predisposed to the development of an incisional hernia. Are there any underlying medical conditions that may predispose to raised intra-abdominal pressure or impaired wound healing? A heavy lifting job may have contributed to the development of an incisional hernia.

EXAMINATION

With the patient fully exposed, after inspection comment on the position of the surgical scar(s) and the swelling caused by the hernia

(Fig. 7.7). If the hernia appears lateral to a midline wound, this may indicate a button-holing through a suture or simply be the result of the way it has expanded. Is the hernia reducible? If so, when the patient lies down and relaxes the hernia will reduce, whereas if asked to cough or tense up the abdominal muscles (by lifting the head off the pillow or raising a straightened leg), the hernia will become obvious. Alternatively the hernia may be incarcerated and impossible to reduce fully. An incarcerated hernia may be covered by red, oedematous skin, suggesting strangulation of the contents – more likely in an emergency surgical patient than in the exam. Attempt to define the neck of the hernia, and determine whether it is wide or narrow.

TREATMENT

After rehydration (with intravenous fluids) and a nasogastric aspiration tube if there is intestinal obstruction, treatment of an incisional hernia, under general anaesthetic, is surgical, by reopening and resuturing the wound and then suturing a mesh over the defect. Remember that the repair of a large incisional hernia can significantly increase intra-abdominal pressure, and lead to respiratory embarrassment.

Fig. 7.7 Incisional hernia.

1 Extent of hernia   **2** Surgical scar   ③ Omentum   ④ Colon   ⑤ Jejunum

Umbilical and paraumbilical hernias

True umbilical hernias occur in infants and are hernias through a weakened umbilical scar. Usually the hernia will improve spontaneously and there is little risk of strangulation.

In adults, hernias around the unbilicus occur, not through the umbilical scar but as a protrusion through the lineas alba just above or below the umbilicus (paraumbilical hernia). These may be relatively small protrusions or large sacs. A common cause of hernia around the umbilicus recently has been laparoscopy, so ensure that you look for any scars.

COMPLICATIONS OF UNTREATED HERNIA

- Pain
- Increasing size
- Ischaemia of contents
- Necrosis of contents
- Death.

COMPLICATIONS OF HERNIA SURGERY

- Early:
  - urinary retention
  - spermatic cord/vascular damage
  - wound infection
  - chest infection
- Late:
  - hernia recurrence
  - testicular atrophy.

Other groin swellings

Lumps in the groin or scrotum can be divided into three categories: scrotal swellings, non–hernia groin lumps and hernias. In addition, palpable lymph nodes and skin lesions (sebaceous cyst, squamous carcinoma of the penis) may occur in this region.

HISTORY

The age and sex of the patient are obviously crucial to the probable diagnosis. The history of the swelling – when it first appeared, whether it is tender, if it has changed in size or shape, whether it can be moved, what structures it is attached to – is indicative of the likely diagnosis. Is there more than one lump? Are the lumps unilateral or bilateral?

Is there a history of trauma, recent exercise or previous surgery (especially hernia or scrotal surgery including vasectomy), or investigation such as femoral artery puncture (particularly for angiography)? Is there a history of sexually transmitted infection?

Past medical history, medications and systematic enquiry should also be documented.

EXAMINATION (Fig. 7.8)

In men, scars in the groin or on the scrotum can be extremely difficult to identify. Compare the two sides; examine the normal side first; check that there are two testes and ask about any scrotal swelling (Fig. 7.9):

Fig. 7.8 Groin and scrotal swellings.

1 Indirect inguinal hernia
2 Femoral hernia
3 Femoral artery aneurysm
4 Lymph nodes
5 Cyst of cord
6 Hydrocele
7 Varicocele
8 Epididymal cyst
9 Testicular cancer
10 Inguinal ligament
11 Femoral artery
12 Femoral vein
13 Pubic tubercle

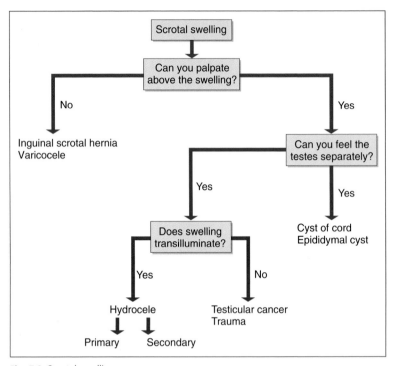

Fig. 7.9 Scrotal swelling.

- Is it tender (leave the tender area to last)?
- Can you feel that the testis is separate from the lump (e.g. epididymal cyst, cyst of the cord or hernia)?
- Can you palpate above the lump? (If so, it may be a true testicular swelling, an epididymal cyst or a hydrocele; if not, it may be an indirect inguinal hernia.)
- Can you transilluminate the lump? (If so, it is fluid filled and likely to be a hydrocele.)
- Male patients should be asked to retract the foreskin (if present) to look for pathologies.

KEY POINT

- Ultrasound examination is very useful to aid diagnosis of scrotal swellings

INVESTIGATION

The key investigation for groin and testicular swellings is ultrasonography, which can clearly delineate the various pathologies. You may be asked about tumour markers (e.g. β–hCG [human chorionic gonadotrophin]) and AFP (α-fetoprotein)) if a testicular cancer is suspected.

Hydrocele* (Fig. 7.10)

A hydrocele is common in surgical finals.

> **KEY POINT**
>
> - A hydrocele may be primary (idiopathic or congenital) or secondary to disease of the testis (testicular cancer, epididymal orchitis)

HISTORY

A hydrocele (Fig. 7.10) is sometimes secondary in response to trauma or an underlying abnormality of the testis. Ask about recent trauma (most common in teenagers) or the development of a unilateral or bilateral swelling, often over several weeks.

Fig. 7.10 Hydrocele.

1 Hydrocele
2 Testis
3 Epididymus
4 Spermatic cord

EXAMINATION

Inspect the difference in size between the two sides, and palpate the hydrocele (Fig 7.10) to differentiate it from the cord, but note that the hydrocele may obscure the testis and epididymus within. A hydrocele can be transilluminated by placing a torch light on to the skin overlying the hydrocele and looking for transilluminated light 'lighting up' the hydrocele.

INVESTIGATION AND TREATMENT

Ultrasonography will demonstrate the hydrocele, testis and epididymus. Treatment, if required, for a primary hydrocele, is by drainage and then suturing the tunica to prevent reaccumulation of the fluid. Treatment for a scondary hydrocele is based on the underlying pathology.

Epididymal cyst*

An epididymal cyst is usually about 1 cm in size, and found at the upper pole of the testis. Epididymal cysts may be single or multiple, unilateral or bilateral, and may be tender.

> **KEY POINT**
>
> - An epididymal cyst (see Fig. 7.8) is palpable separate from the testis

Varicocele**

> **KEY POINT**
>
> - With the patient standing a varicocele resembles a bag of worms

HISTORY

The patient may have noted some lumpiness or abnormal appearance of (or feel a heaviness in) the scrotum.

EXAMINATION

A varicocele (Fig. 7.11) is most obvious when the patient stands – the prominent veins, claimed to resemble a mass of worms, will be

Fig. 7.11 Varicocele.

 Varicocele   ② Testis

apparent. A varicocele is said to be more common on the left side, because of the drainage of the left testicular vein into the left renal vein. As a result of this venous drainage, a varicocele of recent onset may suggest a renal cancer.

INVESTIGATION AND TREATMENT

Investigation of the scrotum and the kidneys by ultrasonography will demonstrate the multiple enlarged veins travelling from the testis proximally around the spermatic cord. The veins can be ligated via an incision in the groin or laparoscopically.

Testicular tumours***

True testicular lumps are likely to be testicular tumours but are uncommon in finals. Testicular tumours may, nevertheless, be discussed as part of the differential diagnosis.

HISTORY

Testicular cancer is most common in the age group 20–40 years (teratoma peak age 25, seminoma peak age 35) as a progressive swelling (Fig. 7.12), which is usually painless and may be associated with a reactive hydrocele.

EXAMINATION

On inspection, compare the left and right sides, looking for a difference in size (Fig. 7.12). Gently palpate the testes, normal side first. On the abnormal side, a palpable firm, symmetrically enlarged testis (or rarely an isolated nodule) may be evident. However, a reactive hydrocele around the testicular cancer may obscure the underlying testis. Clinical features that may be associated with a testicular tumour include gynae-comastia or an abdominal mass of retroperitoneal lymph nodes. The lymphatic drainage of the testes is to the para-aortic nodes as a result of the embryonic intra-abdominal origin of the testes, not to the groin, unlike other structures in the groin.

INVESTIGATION AND TREATMENT

On ultrasonography, the tumour will be evident. An elevated AFP and/or β-hCG may support the diagnosis and can be useful to monitor disease burden. After staging, which includes chest radiography and abdominal CT to look for metastatic disease, surgical resection, radiotherapy and chemotherapy provide a high remission rate.

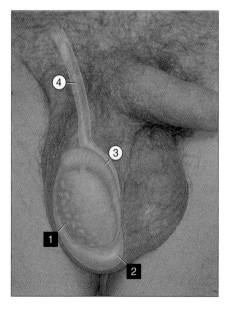

Fig. 7.12 Testicular cancer.

1 Tumour of testis
2 Hydrocele around testis
③ Epididymus
④ Spermatic cord

Ectopic testis***

An ectopic testis is unusual in surgical finals. It is often associated with an inguinal hernia. Beware the absent testis (caused by maldescent, ectopia or surgical removal). Testicular torsion, acutely painful and requiring urgent surgical exploration, does not feature in surgical finals.

Other conditions

The skin of the groin can harbour any of the lumps and bumps described in Chapter 4. Sebaceous cysts are particularly common. Squamous carcinoma of the scrotum, beloved of older textbooks, is no longer a likely short case because the days of the child chimney-sweep are long gone. However, squamous carcinoma of the penis is a possible short case and you *must* examine beneath the foreskin of an uncircumcized man (ask the patient to retract his foreskin, or wear gloves to retract it yourself).

In the perianal area, inspect for papillomas (warts, which are common), an abscess or consequent fistula (if there is recurrent perianal sepsis, think of Crohn's disease), or anal carcinoma (a ragged ulcer with a bloody necrotic discharge).

Regional lymph nodes from the glans, the penile and scrotal skin, and the anus are in the groin. Therefore infection or tumour growth will be reflected in these nodes. The lymphatic drainage from the testes is intra-abdominal to para-aortic nodes.

KEY QUESTIONS

1. What differentiates indirect inguinal, direct inguinal and femoral hernias?
2. What is the difference between an incarcerated and a strangulated hernia?
3. Is a narrow or a wide neck to a hernial sac more dangerous?
4. What is a sliding hernia?
5. How would you distinguish an indirect inguinal hernia in the scrotum from a hydrocele?
6. How would you distinguish an epididymal cyst from a hydrocele?
7. What lesions other than hernias, hydroceles and epididymal cysts can occur in the groin or perineum?
8. Where do the testicular lymph nodes drain to?

8

Limbs (vascular)

In surgical finals it is common for you to be asked to examine a patient's hand or comment on the lower limb. This may require you to think of several different systems, such as cardiovascular, locomotor and neurological systems, during the examination. There are many conditions that you may encounter, but your examination should follow the same general scheme as elsewhere: exposure/position, inspection, palpation, percussion and auscultation. For orthopaedic problems, this may be modified to: exposure/position, look, feel and move. This is simply a different way of performing inspection and palpation. Percussion has a reduced role in the examination of the limbs and back, but auscultation is important in vascular examination. Specific aspects of your examination of a patient will be more important for vascular problems than for orthopaedic problems, and vice versa. This chapter highlights vascular cases, and Chapter 9 looks at orthopaedic problems likely to come up in surgical finals, although this division is somewhat artificial.

HISTORY

You may be asked to 'Examine this woman's hands' or 'What do you think of this man's lower limbs?', which doesn't leave much scope for taking a history. However, you will be able to judge the approximate age of the patient and the gender. It is sometimes hard to miss the heavily nicotine-stained fingers or mouth of a heavy smoker, and you can impress your examiner by mentioning this (if given the chance). If you are permitted to ask questions, after establishing the age and (former) occupation of the patient, ask an open question such as 'What are the problems that brought you into hospital?' or 'What troubles do you get from your hands/legs?'. Specific questions applicable to particular limb problems are outlined in each section below.

EXAMINATION

Exposure/position

Make sure that you can see the whole of the limb that you are supposed to be examining, and the contralateral limb as well. This means that you will probably have to help the patient undress to expose the body parts in which you are interested. Ensure that the patient is then lying (or sitting) comfortably so that you can proceed.

Inspection

Look at the patient's skin for discoloration, signs of trauma (including surgical scars), ulceration and gangrene. Look for deformities, swelling (joint or soft tissue) and muscle wasting. Ask the patient to lift up each limb to ensure that you are not missing something (such as a pressure sore on the heel). You may need to assist the patient, and do ask if the limb is sore before you touch or move it. You will usually be able to compare the limb you have been asked to examine with the contralateral limb, although amputees are a popular choice of patient for some surgical finals.

Palpation

Ask if the limb or joints are painful before you touch the patient, and watch his or her face during the examination to ensure that you are not causing distress. Feel the temperature of the two limbs (using the dorsum of your fingers, which is said to be the most sensitive part), examine the nails and assess capillary filling (blanch the nail with pressure from your finger, then see how long it takes for the colour to return). Palpate the major limb pulses, on the right and left sides.

Auscultation

Auscultation is normally confined to listening for bruits over the arterial tree, but take care that any bruit you hear is not transmitted from more proximal vessels that are diseased. Rarely, arteriovenous malformations may appear in finals. Unless the arteriovenous connection is a surgically manufactured fistula (usually in the forearm, for access for dialysis), and so has a high flow rate, you are unlikely to hear a bruit.

TYPICAL CASES

- Arterial disease:
  - occlusive★
  - aneurysmal★★
  - arteriovenous fistula★★★
- Venous disease:
  - varicose veins★
  - venous thrombosis★★
- Lymphatic disease:
  - primary lymphoedema★★★
  - secondary lymphoedema.★★

Arterial disease*

Chronic arterial insufficiency secondary to atherosclerosis is almost a certainty in surgical finals. The symptoms are usually worse in the lower limbs than in the upper limbs, so patients used in exams usually have lower limb problems. The following scheme for history and examination is presented in terms of the lower limbs, but can easily be modified for use in the context of the upper limbs.

KEY POINTS

- Claudication distance suggests the severity of arterial disease (shorter = more severe)
- The muscle groups affected indicates the likely site(s) of stenosis

---

HISTORY

A general medical history should include a history of smoking (current, previous, never, number of cigarettes) and diabetes, with a note of the type of diabetes and the degree of diabetic control. Ischaemic heart disease, cerebrovascular accidents, hypertension, hypercholesterolaemia, rheumatic heart disease, family history of vascular disease or chronic obstructive pulmonary disease may be associated with lower limb arterial disease. The use of medication is important for control of cardiac disease, hypertension and diabetes.

Ask about the lifestyle effects of arterial disease including how it affects daily living and mobility.

The pain of claudication (pain develops on exercise and is relieved when exercise stops) indicates that the blood supply to the muscle(s) affected is inadequate to cope with exercise. It should be distinguished from sciatic nerve pain, which originates in the buttock, passes down the back of the leg to below the knee, and is associated with pain on raising a straight leg and with possible neurological signs. Ask about claudication distance (the distance at which the pain comes on). This is usually remarkably constant for walking either on the flat or up stairs. Ask whether the claudication distance is increasing, static or decreasing, and how the claudication affects daily living. Using your knowledge of the vascular arterial tree (Fig. 8.1) determine which muscle groups are affected by claudication, to indicate where the stenosis is situated:

- Calf pain indicates stenosis of the superficial femoral/popliteal arteries.
- Thigh and calf pain indicate stenosis of the external iliac artery.
- Buttock, thigh and calf pain indicate stenosis of the external and internal iliac arteries.
- Bilateral lower limb pain indicates stenosis of the aorta.

Determine what treatment(s) the patient and his or her clinicians have tried. Rest pain in a limb is a sign of severe ischaemia, and of impending gangrene, because the arterial perfusion is inadequate even for the skin. Rest pain often occurs first in bed at night, when the limb is warm and perfusion pressure is lowered by the horizontal position – patients may gain relief by dangling the limb over the edge of the bed. This phenomenon can be used in clinical examination (Buerger's test) to assess the time of venous filling/reactive hyperaemia when the leg is dangled over the side of the bed.

EXAMINATION

The limbs to be examined should be fully exposed: for examination of the lower limbs, the patient should wear only underwear from the waist down and, for examination of the upper limbs, no shirt. Remember to expose both limbs so that they can be compared with each other. Patients may be most comfortable lying on a couch (where the lower limbs can readily be seen).

Although they may not obviously be part of an examination of the lower limb, the patient's pulse (rate, rhythm, regularity) and blood pressure (diastolic/systolic) should be recorded as part of a full cardiovascular assessement.

Fig. 8.1 Arteries of the lower limb.

① Common femoral artery   ⑥ Arterial network around knee
② External iliac artery   ⑦ Popliteal artery
③ Internal iliac artery   ⑧ Anterior tibial artery
④ Deep femoral artery   ⑩ Peroneal artery
⑤ Superficial femoral artery ⑪ Dorsalis pedis artery

Look for obvious signs of loss of viability, such as shiny, atrophic skin, hair loss or atrophic nails (the last two are not very specific signs, but should get a mention in exams), ulceration or overt gangrene (Fig. 8.2). Look to see if the limb is pale or has a red, hyperaemic glow and blanches on elevation. Remember to look at the pressure areas (the

Fig. 8.2 Ischaemic lower limbs.

1 Arteriopathic ulcer
2 Gangrenous fifth toe
3 Atrophic skin
4 Hair loss

heel, lateral border of the foot, first metatarsal head and malleoli), particularly in people with diabetes, and look between the toes.

Feel the temperature of the limb (use the dorsum of your fingers) at various levels, and compare it with that of the contralateral limb. Use gentle pressure to check for pitting oedema at the ankle (and more proximally, if it looks oedematous). Assess capillary return in the toe pulp: apply pressure for 2 seconds to blanch the capillary bed, then measure the capillary refill time. Palpate the peripheral pulses: femoral, popliteal (with the patient's knee flexed at 45°, use the pulps of your fingers of both hands to feel for the pulse), dorsalis pedis and posterior tibial (see Fig. 8.1). The scoring convention is: 0 (absent); ± (reduced); 1 (normal); 2 (aneurysmal). Compare the pulses on the left with those on the right. Note the rate, rhythm and regularity, and check for radial/femoral delay.

Listen for bruits over the femoral arteries. Remember that occluded vessels will have no flow, and hence no bruit.

At the end of the history and examination, you should be able to:

- describe the patient's symptoms and signs
- comment on the way in which these affect his or her lifestyle
- say where the vascular tree is occluded.

INVESTIGATION

Test the urine for glucose (diabetes and peripheral vascular disease make a great combined medical and surgical long case) and protein (for renal disease).

Blood should be tested for anaemia or polycythaemia (both of which may worsen the symptoms of peripheral ischaemia), erythrocyte sedimentation rate (ESR; to suggest inflammatory causes of peripheral vascular disease) and biochemistry (to detect renal failure and extent of diabetic control).

An ECG and chest radiograph are useful in the assessment of the general health of patients with peripheral vascular disease, particularly if they are likely to benefit from interventional radiology or reconstructive surgery.

Non-invasive investigations include Doppler scanning, to detect blood flow and measure the pulse pressures, enabling a comparison between the upper limb and lower limb pressures. If Doppler scanning is used to measure the ankle and brachial pressures, the ABPI (ankle/brachial pressure index) can be derived, with the following implications:

ABPI >1.0 – normal
ABPI = 0.7–1.0 – claudication
ABPI = 0.4–0.7 – moderate ischaemia
ABPI <0.4 – severe ischaemia.

Angiography may be considered to be the definitive investigation for arterial disease, because it provides a 'road map' of the patient's vessels, showing the level, length and severity of stenoses and occluded vessels (Fig. 8.3). Angiography is performed by direct arterial puncture (under local anaesthetic) of the femoral artery and, as it is not without potential morbidity (e.g. haematoma, worsening the lower limb ischaemia, embolism of atheromatous plaque to the lower limb), it should be reserved for patients in whom surgical or radiological intervention is contemplated.

Angioscopy, in which the vascular anatomy and abnormalities are directly visualized, is an even more specialized investigation.

MANAGEMENT

The management of lower limb ischaemia may occur over several years and treatment options, as ever, are conservative measures; medical or surgical treatment, and the choice will vary according to the severity of the disease:

Fig. 8.3 Angiogram of lower limb arteries showing atherosclerotic disease and occlusion of the femoral artery.

- Mild/moderate claudication:
  - stop smoking
  - lose weight
  - control diabetes
  - foot care
  - exercise
  - venesection if polycythaemic
  - optimize medical treatment (of diabetes, cardiac function, etc.)
- Disabling claudication:
  - conservative and medical treatment (as above)
  - balloon angioplasty
  - reconstructive surgery
- Critical limb ischaemia:
  - conservative and medical therapy to optimize the patient's general condition
  - balloon angioplasty
  - reconstructive surgery
  - lumbar sympathectomy
  - amputation.

Gangrene*

Dry gangrene (ischaemic), unlike wet gangrene (infective), is a common problem in finals.

The history should be as outlined for peripheral vascular disease. The patient may already have attempted reconstructive vascular surgery or interventional radiology.

On examination, the gangrenous areas may be very small (e.g. the tips of one or more toes), so remember to inspect the heel and between the toes thoroughly. Alternatively, the gangrene may be quite obvious (remember to look at the contralateral limb, which may already have required amputation). Obvious black, hard, gangrenous flesh may be surrounded by skin that is hyperaemic, red and shiny, but still ischaemic (Fig. 8.4).

KEY POINTS

- Dry (ischaemic) gangrene is secondary to peripheral vascular disease
- Wet (infective) gangrene is secondary to bacterial infection

Atrial fibrillation*

The most common abnormal pulse that you will be asked to feel in finals is that associated with atrial fibrillation (AF), although you cannot say so straight away and spoil the examiners' fun! Technically, you

Fig. 8.4 Ischaemic foot.

1 Demarcation of critical ischaemia

2 Atrophic skin

3 Hyperaemia

should also require an ECG, which will demonstrate the absence of P waves and an irregularly irregular pulse. Common causes of AF include ischaemic heart disease, posterior myocardial infarction, hyperthyroidism and rheumatic heart disease.

Acute limb ischaemia**

Although you are unlikely to meet a patient with acute (as opposed to chronic) limb ischaemia, which is a surgical emergency if the limb is to be saved, you may see a patient who has had surgery for acute limb ischaemia or get into a discussion on the topic after seeing a patient with chronic limb ischaemia. The symptoms and signs of acute ischaemia are known as the 'six Ps':

- Pain
- Pulseless
- Pallor
- Perishingly cold (a bit contrived!)
- Paraesthesia
- Powerless.

The first four of these features occur at the time of the acute ischaemic event: either embolic (which may be secondary to AF) or thrombosis on an atherosclerotic plaque, and the neurological effects afterwards.

The aim of treatment is to restore the circulation as soon as possible. If embolic occlusion is suspected, retrieval of the thrombus using a balloon (Fogarty) catheter can be attempted during surgical exploration of the artery, which should be followed by anticoagulation using heparin. If this is unsuccessful, intraoperative angiography is needed. Alternatively, in patients where thrombosis in pre-existing arterial disease is suspected, the key investigation is angiography before surgery, with the option of lysis of the occluding thrombus. Potential complications include recurrence of the ischaemia (and new emboli?), loss of (part of) the limb, compartment syndrome and myoglobin-induced renal failure.

Amputations**

In contrast to upper limb amputations (which are usually traumatic in origin, and often involve one or more digits), amputations of the lower limb are usually surgical and secondary to vascular disease.

Amputations that you may be shown in finals are described below; common amputations are marked with an asterisk:

- Hindquarter: amputation through the hip
- Above knee★ (Fig. 8.5):
  - amputation through the distal femur
  - prosthesis may be fitted
  - less mobility than for below knee
- Through knee: amputation through the knee joint
- Below knee★ (Fig. 8.6):
  - tibia transected 10 cm below the knee joint
  - knee joint retained
  - flexibility and mobility good
- Syme amputation: heel forms the stump: common in nineteenth century as a result of trauma
- Midfoot: through the tarsal/metatarsal junction
- Metatarsal: individual, usually fifth, metatarsal + digit
- Digital★ (Fig. 8.7): one or more digits.

Accompanying the amputation(s), there may be contractures or infected/incompletely healed amputation wounds. The patient may have a walking stick or prosthesis, or even be sitting in a wheelchair; everyday functional living may be achieved with rehabilitation.

Fig. 8.5 Above-knee amputation.

1 Amputation scar
② Femur
③ Superficial femoral artery
④ Deep femoral artery

Fig. 8.6 Below-knee amputation.

1 Amputation scar
2 Scars from contralateral arterial reconstruction
③ Femur
④ Tibia
⑤ Fibula

Fig. 8.7 Digital amputation.

1 Scar from second digit amputation
② Dorsalis pedis artery
③ Arcuate artery
④ Communication with deep plantar artery
⑤ Medial malleolus
⑥ Lateral malleolus

Diabetic foot**

The diabetic patient with lower limb disease may have many of the features already described above. The combination of neuropathy with arterial disease, and perhaps with infection, puts the lower limb (and particularly the foot) at risk. Patients with these conditions are usually comparatively young, with the pulses present and a warm (often infected) foot, and can be contrasted with an older patient with peripheral vascular disease, who has a cold, pulseless foot with dry gangrene.

Peripheral aneurysms***

Trauma (including iatrogenic trauma caused by arterial puncture), atherosclerosis or inflammatory disease can weaken the wall of an artery, resulting in an aneurysm. Although an abdominal aortic aneurysm springs to mind first, you may also encounter in surgical finals a sub-clavian artery aneurysm (which may be associated with thoracic outlet compression), a femoral artery aneurysm (usually at the site of arterial puncture) or a popliteal artery aneurysm.

HISTORY

If you can take a full history as outlined above, all well and good. If you can only ask three questions (e.g. in a short case), ask if there is any history of smoking, diabetes (and preferably how it is controlled) or trauma.

EXAMINATION

Full exposure of the limb is once again important: this may reveal evidence of embolism to, and consequent ischaemia (or gangrene) of, the digits as a result of a subclavian aneurysm, or thrombosis caused by a popliteal aneurysm (with distal ischaemia).

Inspection may reveal obvious pulsation in the line of the subclavian, femoral or popliteal artery. Unfortunately an ectatic artery in a thin, older person can appear at first sight to be an aneurysm (the carotid version of this is unkindly called a 'student's aneurysm' for that very reason). Hence palpation (to demonstrate an expansile lesion, the size of which can be measured) is required to establish the diagnosis.

An audible bruit may be apparent over or distal to the aneurysm, as a result of the disordered flow caused by the aneurysm.

INVESTIGATIONS

Angiography is the key investigation for peripheral aneurysms, but preparation of the patient for theatre will require in addition urinalysis, a full blood count (FBC), blood biochemistry, ECG, chest radiograph, etc. For an aortic aneurysm an ultrasound ± CT scan will be required to determine the relationship of the aneurysm to the renal vessels.

TREATMENT

Conventional surgical treatment usually involves bypassing the affected segment of the vessel, using a vein or synthetic graft, and tying off the aneurysm.

Arteriovenous malformations***

It is possible for an arteriovenous malformation to require an increased cardiac output and hence to cause a hyperdynamic circulation (with an aortic flow murmur), or even heart failure. Alternatively, the result may be limb hypertrophy or ulceration.

HISTORY

The duration of the lesion (has it been present since birth?), any history of trauma (surgical or otherwise) and any change in the size of the lesion or symptoms (e.g. discomfort) related to the malformation are important.

EXAMINATION

Adequately expose the lesion and the remainder of the limb (or torso, if the lesion is there). Inspection should allow you to comment on the position, size (in centimetres), shape, colour and contour of the lesion, and on any associated features such as scars (surgical or traumatic).

Next palpate the lesion for consistency, pulsation, compressibility, draining/filling on raising/lowering the limb, and thrill. Then auscultate for a bruit (a continuous murmur).

Haemangioma***

A haemangioma can range in size from a few millimetres to a large, disfiguring lesion with associated increased growth of the ipsilateral limb, resulting from increased blood flow. A small haemangioma may contain thrombosed blood, and so have a bluish tinge and feel firm. If the outflow is intact, the haemangioma may feel soft and may empty with pressure.

Haemangiomas are not usually fixed to deeper tissues, and rarely have a bruit (but you still need to listen, to please your examiner!).

Arteriovenous fistula***

In exams and hospital practice the common arteriovenous fistula is that which has been formed for dialysis access, usually at the wrist, antecubital fossa or ankle.

There may be visible venous filling (greater on the side with the fistula than on the contralateral side) and there will be a surgical scar, a palpable thrill and, on auscultation, an audible bruit.

Venous disease*

Venous disease and (especially) varicose veins are common in finals, and make particularly good short cases. It will be assumed by every teacher and examiner you meet that you have seen hundreds of patients with varicose veins, so take the trouble to see such patients and examine them under supervision on the wards and in the Outpatient Department.

KEY POINTS

- Varicose veins follow saphenofemoral and venous valve incompetence
- Varicose veins may follow deep venous thrombosis
- Varicose ulceration, consequent upon varicose veins, occurs proximal to the medial malleolus

HISTORY

Questions, in addition to those about the patient's general health and fitness for surgery, should include the onset, distribution and symptoms from the veins. Their onset may be the result of a problem with the deep venous system, so ask about deep venous thrombosis (DVT), pulmonary embolism and trauma to the lower limb. More commonly, varicose veins result from congenital saphenofemoral incompetence or occur during pregnancy. The distribution may sound as though it is related to the long saphenous vein or the short saphenous vein, or perhaps both. Varicose veins often get blamed for all sorts of symptoms to which they are unrelated, but skin itch, ache, bruising and ulceration may be mentioned.

Ask about previous surgery, involving a high tie (saphenofemoral ligation), venous stripping (of the long saphenous vein), multiple ligations or avulsions. Was surgery performed on the short saphenous system? Has there been a second or third operation? Has skin grafting been required for varicose ulceration?

EXAMINATION

Follow the standard exposure/position, inspection, palpation, percussion and (auscultation) scheme.

Having exposed both legs to the groin, varicose veins will be most readily demonstrated with the patient standing (Fig. 8.8). Look at each lower limb in turn, and comment on the distribution of visible varicose veins to the long saphenous system (Fig. 8.9) (from the groin, the vein passes posteromedial to the knee joint, then anterior to the medial malleolus), the distribution of visible varicose veins to the short saphenous system (Fig. 8.10) (from the popliteal fossa, the vein passes inferiorly to the lateral border of the foot), ulceration (typically proximal to the medial malleolus, adjacent to the long saphenous vein) and surgical scars (these can sometimes be difficult to see).

Fig. 8.8 Varicose veins originating from the long saphenous system.

Fig. 8.9 Normal anatomy of the long saphenous vein.

① Long saphenous vein
② Saphenofemoral junction
③ Common sites of incompetent perforating veins
④ Medial malleolus
⑤ Patella

Varicose ulcers (Fig. 8.11) should be differentiated from arteriopathic, neuropathic, diabetic, vasculitic (particularly rheumatoid), infective (e.g. syphilitic) and malignant ulcers. Arterial ulcers are usually sited on the lateral border of the lower limb, proximal to the lateral malleolus (i.e. furthest from the dorsalis pedis and posterior tibial arteries) (Table 8.1).

Use palpation to confirm what you suspect from inspection. Remember to check both sides, because the limbs may have a different distribution of varicose veins. With the patient still standing, start proximally and confirm that the soft (bluish) reducible swelling over the saphenofemoral junction (just medial to the femoral artery if you are in any

Fig. 8.10 Normal anatomy of the short saphenous vein.

① Short saphenous vein
② Popliteal vein
③ Biceps femoris muscle
④ Semitendinosus muscle
⑤ Gastrocnemius muscle

Fig. 8.11 Varicose ulcer.

1 Ulcer
2 Lipodermosclerosis
3 Healed ulcer
④ Medial malleolus

doubt), which has a fluid thrill when the patient coughs and empties on direct pressure, is a saphenous varix. Palpate the soft, but firm, varicose veins. You may be able to feel defects in the fascia – one a (patient's) hand-breadth proximal to the knee joint, one distal to the knee joint and one proximal to the medial malleolus. These may

Table 8.1 Common lower limb ulcers

	Venous	**Ischaemic**	**Trophic**	**Malignant**
Site	Lower calf, typically superior to medial malleolus	Dorsum of foot over pressure points	Pressure points, i.e. over metatarsals	May relate to venous ulcer or other scars
Associated conditions	Varicose veins	Atherosclerosis	Diabetic neuropathy	Bowen's disease
	Previous DVTs	Loss of peripheral pulses	Peripheral vascular disease	
		Rheumatoid disease		
Edge of ulcer	Shelving	Shelving	'Punched out' Deep	'Heaped' or everted
Base of ulcer	Frequently moist slough	Slough with poor granulation	Often dry eschar but may extend to bone	Frequently moist slough
Surrounding skin	Varicose eczema Liposclerosis	Thin and atrophic	May be normal	Dependent upon predisposing conditions

represent the sites of incompetent perforators from the deep to the superficial systems.

Percuss the column of blood in the great saphenous vein with one hand, while feeling with the other further proximally.

Trendelenburg's test

To determine the level of incompetent perforators:

1. Lie the patient on a couch, elevate the lower limb and empty the varicose veins.
2. Tighten a tourniquet around the upper thigh, hold the tourniquet in position and ask the patient to stand.

3. If saphenofemoral incompetence is the sole cause of the varicosities, the varicose veins will not fill until you release the tourniquet 5 seconds later (when the veins fill rapidly). If the veins fill before the tourniquet is released, there are other incompetent (perforator) veins distally.
4. Repeat the process – lie the patient down, empty the veins, apply the tourniquet distal to the site of the potentially incompetent perforator, stand the patient up and look for varicosity filling before the tourniquet is released.
5. Continue until all the perforators have been identified.

Remember to feel for the peripheral arterial pulses if there is an ulcer: it could be an ischaemic ulcer, even if the patient has varicose veins.

INVESTIGATIONS

In addition to the basic investigations for the assessment of a patient's fitness for anaesthesia (blood biochemistry and haematology, ECG and chest radiology where appropriate), further investigation of the varicose veins is advisable if they are recurrent (to identify the incompetent perforators) or if there is a previous history of DVT or lower limb trauma, to ensure that there is an intact deep venous system.

Doppler scanning (Fig. 8.12) for venous blood flow through incompetent valves (i.e. from the high-pressure deep venous system to the low-pressure superficial veins) can be used to identify the incompetent perforator veins, which may be sited at the classic positions. Alternatively, ascending venography can be used to map out the venous anatomy of the lower limb in complicated cases, particularly if the integrity of the deep venous system is in doubt (e.g. following a previous DVT).

MANAGEMENT

Conservative measures include the use of graduated compression stockings. Medical treatment does not have a role, but there are several surgical options. These range from injection sclerotherapy (for small veins distal to the knee), laser therapy (for small venous flares) and local ligation under local anaesthetic, to the standard high tie (saphenofemoral junction ligation) and the multiple ligation or avulsion of more distal vessels – to which may be added the stripping out of the long saphenous

Fig. 8.12 Varicose veins from short saphenous system. Doppler probe and calf compression in use to show site of deep to superficial incompetence (marked X).

① Short saphenous vein
② Popliteal vein
③ Semitendinosus muscle
④ Biceps muscle
⑤ Gastrocnemius muscle
6 Incompetent popliteal/short saphenous communicating
7 Varicosities

vein from the groin to just distal to the knee, to reduce the chance of recurrence.

The swollen limb**

A swollen limb may be upper or lower, unilateral or bilateral, and result from general or localized problems. General problems causing bilateral lower limb swelling include cardiovascular causes (e.g. cardiac failure), renal causes (e.g. nephrotic syndrome) and low-protein states (e.g. hypoalbuminaemia). Local problems (which may cause unilateral or bilateral swelling of the lower limb) can be categorized as venous obstruction (e.g. DVT), lymphatic obstruction or intra-abdominal or intrathoracic obstruction of the venous or lymphatic systems. Lower limb swelling is more common in surgical finals than is upper limb swelling, which is comparatively rare except in patients with treated breast cancer.

Deep venous thrombosis**

> ### KEY POINTS
>
> - Predisposing factors: immobility, trauma, malignancy
> - Occurs 7–10 days postoperatively
> - Symptoms of pulmonary embolism

HISTORY

Ask how long the limb has been swollen, in what circumstances the swelling was first noted and whether the limb is painful. The recent history should include questions about predisposing factors such as recent surgery (particularly hip, knee or intra-abdominal surgery), immobility, trauma to the limb or pelvis, malignancy and medications (particularly the oral contraceptive pill and oestrogen-containing preparations). A past history of DVT or pulmonary embolism (PE) is important. The patient may tell you what medications he or she has been or is taking (heparin? warfarin?). Ask about respiratory symptoms, thinking of PE, particularly sharp (pleuritic) chest pain on inspiration, haemoptysis or breathlessness. Typically, DVT becomes clinically apparent a few days postoperatively and PE appears 7–10 days postoperatively.

Long-term sequelae of DVT may be the development of 'post-thrombotic syndrome', characterized by chronic limb swelling, dilated veins, varicose eczema and ulceration.

EXAMINATION

Expose the lower limbs up to the groin, with the patient lying comfortably on a bed or couch. Is there a pump administering heparin (the name of the drug should be written on the syringe or bag)? Look at the distribution of the swelling: is it unilateral or bilateral, and how far proximally does it extend up each limb? For a more objective test, measure the circumference of the calf and that of the thigh 10 cm below the tibial tuberosity and 10 cm above the top of the patella respectively. Compare them with those of the opposite side. Are the classic signs of a red, swollen limb with shiny skin and visible superficial veins apparent (Fig. 8.13) (not all features may be present)?

Having asked the patient whether the limb is tender (and if so, where the tenderness is), gently compare the temperature of the two limbs using the dorsum of your fingers: the side with the DVT should be

Fig. 8.13 Unilateral (left) deep venous thrombosis.

warmer. With gentle pressure, elicit pitting oedema. Homan's sign (dorsiflexion of the ankle to elicit calf pain) is a very non-specific sign of DVT, and many clinicians would not encourage you to use it. Gentle palpation of the calf and over the adductor canal may elicit discomfort in a patient with DVT.

You should ask to go on to examine the respiratory system if you suspect a PE (listen particularly for a localized pleural rub over the infarcted lung).

Percussion or auscultation of the limb is not helpful.

INVESTIGATIONS

As the symptoms and signs of a DVT or PE are non-specific, a high index of clinical suspicion, based on the patient's history, may be all that you have to suggest the diagnosis. The radiology and medical physics departments carry out the key investigations.

Doppler scanning, to detect blood flow in the deep veins of the lower limb, is non-invasive but less specific than ascending venography, which can outline the veins containing thrombus and demonstrate collateral pelvic vessels (Fig. 8.14). Techniques using radioisotopes to detect thrombus are in vogue in some centres.

In the case of PE, the radiological features on a chest film may be non-specific, simply showing small segmental defects. Similarly, the ECG appearances of changes in the S wave in lead I, and changes in the Q and T waves in lead III, are not diagnostic. However, a perfusion scan may show segmental defects and, when combined with a ventilation scan (to show ventilation–perfusion mismatch), will indicate the probability (low, medium or high) that PE has occurred. Pulmonary angiography, although rarely performed, is the definitive investigation. Increasing use of spiral CT may mean that it may soon become the investigation of choice.

MANAGEMENT

Conservative measures for the prevention of DVT include the use of graduated compression stockings, pneumatic compression boots and early postoperative mobility. Medical prevention may include the use of subcutaneous injections of heparin.

Fig. 8.14 Venogram demonstrating right common iliac vein thrombus and collateral venous drainage.

Formal treatment of DVT is aimed at preventing the extension or detachment of a segment of thrombus, and hence PE. Treatment comprises intravenous heparin infusion (some authorities recommend subcutaneous heparin injection as an alternative) with conversion to oral warfarin after 3 days, to maintain a therapeutic level of anticoagulation for 3–6 months. A vena caval filter may be indicated for patients with recurrent thromboembolism (from the lower limb or pelvic veins) despite adequate anticoagulation.

Lymphatic disease**

Lymphoedema may be primary (failure of the lymphatics to develop – more likely in the lower limbs (Fig. 8.15) than the upper limbs, and comparatively rare) or secondary (caused by mechanical obstruction of the lymphatics, as a result of a disease process or of surgical or radiotherapy treatment).

A lymphoedematous limb is particularly prone to sepsis, so a patient has to be aware of the potential problems (e.g. cellulitis and

Fig. 8.15 Bilateral lymphoedema of lower limbs.

lymphangitis) that may arise from even quite minor abrasions. Rarely, a sarcoma may develop in the axilla of a lymphoedematous limb.

HISTORY

Patients in surgical finals with lymphoedema are likely to have had a tumour or treatment for a cancer involving the surgical excision of regional nodes, or radiotherapy to the regional nodes. The most likely cause of upper limb oedema is breast cancer (because of tumour infiltration, or surgery or radiotherapy to the axilla). In the case of the lower limb, intra-abdominal causes (particularly tumours) are likely for bilateral oedema (if one excludes cardiovascular disease and hypoproteinaemia), and one likely cause of unilateral lymphoedema is dissection of groin nodes (e.g. in melanoma).

In a long case, make sure that you ascertain a clear sequence of events and treatments: often the patient will be quite helpful.

EXAMINATION

With the limb in question and the contralateral limb exposed, look for surgical scars or signs of radiotherapy and compare the two sides. In the case of the upper limb, remember to inspect the chest wall for signs of treated or advanced breast cancer. Look to see whether the patient is wearing a compression stocking or armlet, or whether this is nearby. A graduated compression boot or sleeve, which uses a pump, may also be nearby.

Before palpation, ask whether the limb is tender or sore anywhere. Avoid tender areas. Gentle palpation will distinguish between a pitting oedema and a chronic, woody, non-pitting oedema.

Percussion or auscultation is not likely to be helpful.

INVESTIGATION

The investigation of lymphoedema should be aimed at discovering the cause. This may be self-evident from the history and inspection (e.g. a patient with breast cancer treated by mastectomy, axillary node clearance and radiotherapy).

TREATMENT

If a tumour is causing obstruction of the lymphatics, radiotherapy may result in reduction of the lymphoedema. However, upper limb lymphoedema is usually secondary to radiotherapy or surgery (or both) in the axilla and will rarely improve with (further) radiotherapy, so treatment is aimed at trying to minimize the swelling by using an arm stocking and preventing infection.

KEY QUESTIONS

1. What are the features of claudication?
2. What are the signs of arterial insufficiency of the lower limb in:
   - acute ischaemia?
   - chronic ischaemia?
3. How does the presentation of acute limb ischaemia differ from that of chronic arterial occlusion?
4. How would you investigate a patient with claudication?
5. What is the significance of rest pain in a patient with peripheral vascular disease, and how should this be managed?
6. What is the difference between wet gangrene and dry gangrene?
7. Are the following true or false?
   - Arteriovenous malformations may cause excessive limb growth.
   - The brachial artery is in danger from supracondylar humeral fractures.
8. What are the predisposing factors for varicose veins?
9. How would you examine a patient with varicose veins?
10. How would you investigate and treat a patient with DVT?
11. What are the long-term sequelae of DVT?
12. What are the likely causes and complications of unilateral upper limb oedema?

9

Limbs (locomotor) and back

Patients with orthopaedic problems make good short cases from the examiners' point of view, because they test your knowledge of basic anatomy, your clinical examination and whether you have attended the orthopaedic part of your clinical attachments. A long case patient may have multiple medical problems as well as the principal condition (e.g. rheumatoid arthritis with cardiovascular and renal disease), which you may need to consider. Follow the now familiar scheme of history and examination. The scheme of inspection, palpation, percussion and auscultation is modified for orthopaedic patients to:

- look
- feel
- move.

THE LIMBS

HISTORY

The key areas to ask about include a history of trauma, analgesia and other medications, and orthopaedic operations. Questions should also be asked about the everyday functioning of the patient (e.g. stiffness, mobility, functional grip, walking, pain). Additional medical problems can, as for patients with vascular disease, influence the management options available.

EXAMINATION

Look

Begin your inspection with observation of the patient's posture and, if you are permitted to watch the patient walk (unusual in a surgical exam), of his or her gait. Look for kyphosis, scoliosis, obvious deformities of the limbs (perhaps from a stroke resulting in upper and lower limb deficits) and facial paralysis.

Feel

Having washed your hands, gently palpate visible lumps, contractures, joint line tenderness and effusions (particularly at the knee).

Move

Assess the active movement of joints, including the range of movement (ask the patient to flex or extend the joint), before you proceed to test passive movement. Once again, ensure that you are not causing pain.

Test for motor power, reflexes and sensation, particularly if you think that there is likely to be an abnormality.

TYPICAL CASES

Fractures**

You are very unlikely to see a patient with an acute fracture in your exam, but it is not uncommon for you to be faced with a patient with a treated fracture and to be examined on the initial and subsequent management of this patient. Remember that there may also be significant soft tissue injury. Of particular importance are injuries to adjacent neurovascular structures, and these must be looked for carefully at the time of injury.

KEY POINTS

- Mechanism of injury
- Functional effects
- Related soft tissue injuries

HISTORY

Ask about how the fracture (defined as loss of bone continuity) occurred, the mechanism of the injury (e.g. falling onto an outstretched hand for a Colles' fracture), and whether there was a single injury or multiple trauma (perhaps in a road traffic accident). Was the fracture simple or compound (in which the skin or epithelium overlying the fracture is breached, increasing the risk of sepsis)? Ask about predisposing factors such as osteoporosis, previous injury, previous surgery and previous malignant disease (thinking particularly of bone metastases).

How was the fracture managed? Ask about the analgesia required, the method of anaesthesia, the method of reduction and fixation (manipulation and closed reduction, or open surgery – with or without wires, screws or prostheses), and whether antibiotics or anti-tetanus were given prophylactically.

EXAMINATION

Ensure that you have adequately exposed the limb bearing the fracture, acknowledging that this may be quite difficult if a plaster of Paris (or more modern substitute) is in place, and make sure that the patient is positioned comfortably.

Describe what you can see: this sounds obvious, but it is easy to forget to describe the presence of a plaster or an external fixation device, an obvious deformity, muscle wasting, skin discoloration, loss of skin, scars (surgical or traumatic) or swelling. Comment on whether a joint appears to be involved. Remember to compare the injured limb with the contralateral limb.

Ask if the limb is painful at any site. Feel the temperature of the injured limb, and feel for swelling, pitting oedema, bony discontinuity or protrusions. Feel whether a joint is likely to be involved.

Ask the patient to move the limb (active movement), to determine the range of movement compared with that of the contralateral limb, and the ease of movement. By passive movement of the limb, determine whether there is any abnormal movement (there is unlikely to be bony crepitus in an exam patient, but there may be malunion). Remember that a plaster may obstruct the full range of active or passive movement.

INVESTIGATIONS

Patients needing surgery, particularly elderly people or patients with multiple trauma, will require haematology, blood biochemistry, ECG and chest radiology, but the key investigation for a patient with a fracture is radiology. This must include two views and the joint proximal to and the joint distal to the fracture.

Describe the fracture as far as you can, including the following:

- Type and location of fracture (e.g. a simple/compound fracture of the mid-tibia)
- Pattern of the fracture (e.g. transverse/spiral/comminuted (multiple fragments))
- The deformity (e.g. displacement/angulation/rotation)
- Predisposing factors
- Complicating factors.

Angulation should be described in terms of the direction in which the distal fragment is tilted (e.g. a Colles' fracture of the wrist, with radial and dorsal tilt).

Certain fractures (e.g. of the scaphoid) only really show up at a later date, on a radioisotope bone scan.

TREATMENT

The treatment of any fracture should aim to restore the continuity of the bone and return the patient to full mobility with the minimum of delay. However, fracture treatment may have to take second place in the multiply injured patient, in whom immediate life-saving measures take precedence over the perhaps more dramatic fracture. Always remember that priority must be given to:

- A for **a**irway, with cervical spine control
- B for **b**reathing
- C for **c**irculation (fracture stabilization, with an external splint, may reduce blood loss).

Specific fracture treatment can be summarized as:

1. Initial splinting of the fracture and analgesia.
2. Cleaning and removal of devitalized tissue (débridement) if compound.
3. Reduction of significant deformity.
4. Maintenance of reduction until there is sound bony union.
5. Intervention in response to any complicating factors, such as vascular impairment, if necessary.
6. Full rehabilitation.

There are many different types of fracture and you are unlikely to be asked details about the management of specific individual fractures. Fracture treatment can range from analgesia and a sling (e.g. clavicle), through to a plaster cast (Colles' fracture), internal fixation (femur), external fixation (tibia), hemiarthroplasty (hip) or total joint replacement (hip). The following fractures are sometimes encountered in surgical finals, and illustrate the general principles of fracture management.

Colles' fracture**

- Site: within 2.5 cm of the wrist joint
- Cause: fall on the outstretched hand
- Associated features: osteoporosis (common in elderly women)
- Deformity:
  - dorsal and radial displacement
  - dorsal tilt of distal fragment
- Treatment:
  - manipulation if >10° of angulation
  - plaster from metacarpophalangeal (MCP) joint to below elbow
- Complications: stiffness at wrist:
  - possibility of frozen shoulder caused by enforced immobility of upper limb
  - persisting deformity (e.g. malunion)
  - carpal tunnel syndrome
  - Sudeck's atrophy.

Fractured neck of femur** (Fig. 9.1)

- Site: intracapsular (e.g. subcapital, transcervical)/extracapsular (e.g. intertrochanteric, subtrochanteric)
- Cause, e.g. even apparently minor fall in elderly women

Fig. 9.1 Radiograph of the pelvis showing a fracture of the neck of the right femur.

- Associated features: this is generally a fracture associated with osteoporosis in elderly people
- Deformity: clinically the limb is shortened and externally rotated
- Treatment: usually by internal fixation: this allows early mobilization and minimizes the risk of non-union
- Complications: patients with these fractures are frequently elderly and susceptible to hypostatic pneumonia, bed sores, urinary infections, deep venous thrombosis, pulmonary embolus and muscle wasting if left immobile for a long time. Avascular necrosis of the femoral head is more likely with intracapsular fractures. Non-union may occur if the diagnosis is delayed, or fixation is inadequate.

Rheumatoid arthritis*

There are several aspects of rheumatoid arthritis which you may encounter in either surgical or medical finals. In surgery, you are most likely to be asked to comment on a patient's hands, a rheumatoid nodule or a specific joint as a short case. Occasionally you may encounter a patient with rheumatoid arthritis in your long case, in which event you will have to determine: the features of the arthropathy; systemic features of the disease; treatment already received; planned future management; and other (unrelated) conditions.

Rheumatoid arthritis is usually symmetrical, typically affecting the following joints in middle-aged women: metacarpalphalangeal (MCP), proximal interphalangeal (PIP), wrist, elbow, hip, knee, ankle, metatarsophalangeal and cervical.

KEY POINTS

- Multiple joints symmetrically affected
- Effects on function
- Systemic manifestations

HISTORY

Ask about the features of the arthropathy: the joints affected, the timescale of the disease, the severity of acute exacerbations and the baseline disease. Typically patients will complain of pain and/or loss of function. With loss of function, in particular, you should determine what impact this has on your patient's lifestyle, i.e. can the patient dress him- or herself and cope with day-to-day activities? Does he or she use adapted or special appliances?

Many treatments for rheumatoid arthritis have significant side effects, so ask about both what treatments have been prescribed previously and what is currently being used. Ask about drug treatments and their side effects, e.g. non-steroidal anti-inflammatory drugs (NSAIDs) and dyspepsia, steroids and metabolic disturbances, dyspepsia and weight gain. This being surgical finals, be sure to document any operations that have already been performed.

Rheumatoid arthritis is a systemic autoimmune disease, and you should ask the patient about any extra-articular symptoms suggestive of Sjögren syndrome (dry eyes and mouth, parotid swelling), vasculitis (unusual rashes or leg ulcers), anaemia, renal failure, amyloidosis, sensory neuropathy or Felty syndrome (rheumatoid arthritis, splenomegaly and pancytopenia).

EXAMINATION

Whether you are approaching a patient for the long case or a short case, take a moment to look for a walking stick, walking frame or wheelchair.

Examination should start with observation of the patient's gait, although, in a short case, when you ask if you can stand the patient up and see him or her walk, this may be considered unnecessary by the examiner. On inspection of the exposed hands and forearms (note how the patient undresses), look to see how the patient moves the hands. Are they obviously painful or limited in movement? Ask the patient to show you the palms and then the dorsa of the hands. Look for surgical scars (e.g. from synovectomy, hip, knee and digital joint replacements, joint stabilization) and for rheumatoid nodules. Rheumatoid nodules are subcutaneous masses, usually on the forearm or over the olecranon, that are typical of rheumatoid arthritis. You should treat the nodules as any other lumps that you are asked to examine: describe their size, position, shape, degree of fixation (they will be mobile) and consistency (soft), and additional features (in this case the presence of rheumatoid arthritis). Look at the skin (is it atrophic? is there erythema or bruising?) and look for signs of muscle wasting.

The typical deformity in rheumatoid arthritis of the hands is ulnar deviation and subluxation at the MCP joints. An acute exacerbation will be painful, and there may be swelling and erythema of the affected joints. Rheumatoid arthritis tends to affect the MCP and proximal interphalangeal (PIP) joints rather than the distal interphalangeal (DIP) joints, which are more likely to be affected by osteoarthritis. Look for specific deformities (Fig. 9.2), particularly the boutonnière and swan-neck deformities of the fingers, and the Z deformity of the thumb.

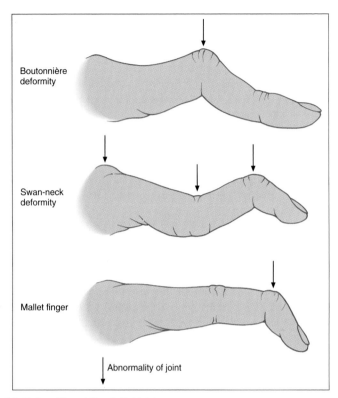

Boutonnière deformity

Swan-neck deformity

Mallet finger

Abnormality of joint

Fig. 9.2 Deformities of the digital joints.

Ask if there are any tender areas, and avoid palpating these if possible. Gently feel the temperature of the skin overlying the joints, and palpate the soft tissue around the joint and the nodules.

Ask the patient to demonstrate the range of active movement that he or she has. Test the range of passive movement and then the power of each limb. Often, rheumatoid arthritic hands are used to test you in the exam, so remember to test pinch grip and the interossei.

INVESTIGATIONS

As rheumatoid arthritis may have multiple systemic manifestations, it is not surprising that a full blood count (FBC) may show anaemia (or pancytopenia in Felty syndrome) and that the erythrocyte sedimentation rate (ESR) may be very high in active disease. Blood biochemistry may provide evidence of renal compromise (as a result of the disease itself or secondary to drug therapy).

After your examination, you may be asked to comment on limb or cervical radiographs. There is a progression of findings as the disease process develops: narrowing of the joint space, osteoporosis, lytic lesions in the periarticular bone, deformity resulting from subluxation of the joint, and finally secondary osteoarthritis. In the cervical spine laxity of the atlantoaxial ligaments and odontoid peg may lead to cord compression and so cervical spine radiographs are essential before any general anaesthetics.

MANAGEMENT

Conservative management of rheumatoid arthritis includes physiotherapy and splintage to avoid deformity, together with drug therapy. Surgery may have a role to remove thickened, inflamed synovium (synovectomy), stabilize unstable joints (arthrodesis), relieve disability and improve function in a destroyed joint (arthroplasty) and treat related soft tissue lesions such as tendon repairs and nerve decompressions.

Osteoarthritis

Whereas rheumatoid arthritis is an autoimmune disease, involving synovial joints, osteoarthritis can be regarded as being caused by wear and tear and so is more common in weight-bearing joints, particularly the hips and knees. Anything that increases the stress on a joint may predispose to osteoarthritis, particularly: obesity, previous fracture with persisting deformity, fracture through a joint, congenital deformities, rheumatoid arthritis, hard manual labour (e.g. miners) and sport.

Osteoarthritis of the hip**

KEY POINTS

- Pain and effects on daily activity
- Walking aids
- Limb shortening, deformities, muscle wasting
- Range of movement
- Muscle power

HISTORY

Ask the patient about pain in the hip, which is often worse on weight bearing, particularly on rising, but may wake the patient at night, when the muscles are relaxed. You should also ask about mobility and any loss of function – particularly, how this interferes with the patient's lifestyle and the use of any appliances at home. Find out about any predisposing factors, such as previous injuries, slipped epiphysis in adolescence or use of steroids (e.g. thinking of avascular necrosis of the femoral head).

EXAMINATION

Examination of the hip should start with observation of the patient's gait. In practice, in an exam situation this is probably best left until the end of the examination – at the beginning, the patient will probably be on a couch awaiting your attention. Ask if you can stand the patient up and see him or her walking, explaining that you will be looking for the typical antalgic gait associated with a painful hip. Nine times out of ten your examiner will say this is not necessary. Check that the patient is lying comfortably (with one pillow), wearing the minimum of clothing from the waist down to preserve modesty but not hinder inspection or further examination. Ensure that the anterosuperior iliac spines are level.

Look to see whether there is a walking stick or walking frame next to the patient. If there is, ask the patient whether he or she uses it. (This checks that it belongs to the patient and makes the examiner, if present, aware that you have spotted it.)

Start by assessing the resting position of the lower limb for shortening, rotation or flexion contractures, look for any scars from previous surgery and comment on any muscle wasting (most marked in the quadriceps and gluteal muscles). In osteoarthritis of the hip, apparent shortening of the lower limb can be detected by measuring the distance from the anterosuperior iliac spine to the medial malleolus on each side. Measuring from the anterosuperior iliac spine to the greater trochanter will demonstrate whether any difference is caused by shortening of the hip joint. Apparent shortening, resulting from flexion deformities and adduction, will be evident on measuring from the umbilicus to each medial malleolus. A fixed flexion deformity may be evident if, in the resting position, the patient's thigh is not in contact with the examination couch – this can be confirmed using Thomas' test (see below). At rest, external rotation of the lower limb (detected most easily by examining the position of the foot at rest) may be evident.

Palpation of the hip joint itself is difficult. Ask if there is any tenderness, then feel for increased temperature and gently palpate the hip.

Test active movement: ask the patient to flex then extend the hip, to adduct then abduct the lower limb and to rotate the hip internally then externally. You need to give precise instructions, and beware of the patient cheating.

Passive movement will allow you to assess fully a fixed flexion deformity. Use Thomas' test: flex the contralateral hip fully (to flatten out the lumbar lordosis) – any flexion at the hip under scrutiny is caused by a fixed flexion deformity in the hip.

Next, passively adduct then abduct the lower limb. Abduction and adduction should be tested with the pelvis fixed in a stationary position. With the patient lying on his or her back, ask him or her to dangle the contralateral leg over the side of the bed. Now place one hand over a line between the two anterosuperior iliac spines and abduct the leg from the midline. When there is tilting of the pelvis (detected by your hand across the two anterosuperior spines), the limit of abduction at the hip has been reached. Note that further abduction is possible by tilting the pelvis, hence fixation of the pelvis during testing.

Passively rotate the hip internally then externally, noting the range of movement and whether there is any pain on movement. Internal and external rotation should be tested with the hip and knee both flexed to 90°, to test true rotation at the hip.

Remember that movement may be limited by pain and, if the patient is sore after a certain range of movement, do not attempt to move the leg even more.

Compare the range of movement in the two hip joints. Ideally a goniometer should be used to measure the range of movement in each direction for each hip. For each aspect of movement (flexion, extension, etc.), test power using the following grading system:

0 – no movement
1 – visible muscle contraction, no joint movement
2 – joint movement when gravity eliminated
3 – movement overcomes gravity
4 – movement overcomes gravity and resistance
5 – normal power.

INVESTIGATION

After the history and examination, you will often be shown the patient's radiographs. Hopefully the patient will have a relatively normal contralateral hip with which to compare the abnormal one, but this is by no means certain. As in rheumatoid disease, there is a progression of changes in osteoarthritis as follows: loss of joint space; osteosclerosis in the periarticular bone; cyst and osteophyte formation in the bone adjacent to the joint; and finally, collapse of the femoral head and the acetabular roof.

MANAGEMENT

Initial conservative management will include advice on weight loss, the use of a walking stick and NSAIDs. As pain and disability increase, there is a growing indication for total hip replacement, which has the twin benefits of restoring function and reducing pain. Occasionally an intertrochanteric osteotomy may be utilized to shift the stresses placed on an arthritic hip but this is far less common than a total hip replacement.

Osteoarthritis of the knee**

KEY POINTS

- Pain and functional effects on daily activity
- Deformities, effusions and muscle wasting
- Range of movement

HISTORY

Ask the patient about pain and stiffness in the knee joint and about how his or her lifestyle is affected. The patient may have noticed swelling or occasional locking of the knee (commonly associated with cartilage tears, but sometimes caused by loose bodies). You should also ask about any predisposing causes of the arthritis, particularly trauma, sporting activities and previous orthopaedic operations. Although difficulty with stairs may more commonly be a feature of ligamentous injury (particularly of the cruciates) than of osteoarthritis, you should ask about walking up and down stairs: is there any apprehension or sense of the knee being about to 'give way'?

EXAMINATION

Many of the steps in the examination of the osteoarthritic knee, or any other problematic knee, are similar to those for the examination of the hip. Expose the entirety of both lower limbs.

Inspect the whole leg, and then the knee. Are there any scars? Does it appear swollen? Is there any obvious deformity of the joint (valgus or varus)? Is there any muscle wasting, particularly of vastus medialis? Ideally, you should see the patient walk, to assess the gait, and watch the patient walk up and down stairs.

Before you touch the limb, ask if it is tender anywhere. Use the dorsa of your fingers to check the temperature of the knee, and compare it with that of the other side. Measure the circumference of the left and right thighs at the same distance (10 cm) proximal to the knee joint, to confirm any subjective impression of muscle wasting. With the knee flexed at 30–45°, palpate the patella and around its margins, then feel the lower femur, the tibia and the head of the fibula: comment on any tenderness or abnormal bony projections (most likely to be osteophytes). Remember to palpate along the medial and lateral cartilages, and over the origin and insertion of the collateral ligaments and popliteal fossa.

Test for an effusion. Place one hand on the thigh and empty out the suprapatellar bursa. With that hand kept in place, gently compress the inner aspect of the knee at the hollow behind the patella, and as you do this watch the other side of the knee to see if there is any bulging (suggesting fluid). If you are unsure, repeat the procedure but stroke the outer aspect as you watch the inner aspect. A patellar tap is a good method of detecting a moderate or large effusion: empty the suprapatellar bursa, then use your other hand to demonstrate a springy tap by pressing sharply on the patella.

The movements of the knee are flexion and extension, with some rotation to lock the knee at the extreme of extension. As always, test active movements before progressing to passive movements. Comment on the range of movement and power (graded 0–5 – see page 231) of the muscle groups.

Although it is unlikely to be useful in examination of the osteoarthritic knee, in other circumstances you may wish to test for any ligamentous laxity (medial and lateral collateral ligaments) and for anterior or posterior cruciate tears. To examine for collateral ligament laxity: with the lower limb almost fully extended (but the knee not locked), push one hand against the medial side of the knee to test for lateral collateral ligament laxity and vice versa. To examine for cruciate disruption (which may be evident only in the presence of collateral ligament disruption): flex the knee to 90°, fix the foot and, with the hamstring muscles relaxed, use two hands placed behind the upper tibia to test for the anterior drawer sign (anterior cruciate disruption) by attempting to pull the tibia towards you. Then, by pushing the tibia away from you, test for posterior cruciate laxity.

You are unlikely to be asked to perform the apprehension test (for patellar instability) or the McMurray test (for a torn meniscus) in surgical finals.

INVESTIGATION

After your examination of the knee, ask to inspect radiographs of the knee joint. The radiological signs of osteoarthritis of the knee are similar to those of osteoarthritis of the hip: narrowed joint space, osteosclerosis, and subcartilagenous cyst and osteophyte formation.

MANAGEMENT

As for osteoarthritis of the hip, initial medical management includes NSAIDs and lifestyle changes. Total knee replacement may be required as the joint becomes increasingly arthritic.

Peripheral nerve lesions*

These are much beloved by examiners as short cases – it gives them a chance to observe you examining, and also an opportunity to test your long-forgotten knowledge of anatomy. Peripheral nerve lesions are more likely to appear in a surgical exam than are general neuropathies (e.g. as seen in people with diabetes or alcoholic problems, or as side effects of drugs, and in patients with primary neurological diseases). It is important in surgical finals to know the sensory distribution and motor function of the major peripheral nerves. Contrast these with the sensory distribution of the nerve roots and the muscles supplied by them: it can all become quite complex. Figure 9.3 shows a diagrammatical way of remembering some of the key points.

> **KEY POINT**
>
> - Knowledge of the site of injury and of the sensory and motor distributions of a nerve will allow you to predict the functional effects

HISTORY

Ask about any history of trauma, the distribution of pain or paraesthesia, and any weakness. Enquire about the functional use of the limb in question, both in everyday life and at work. Ask whether any surgery

Sensory	Power	Reflexes
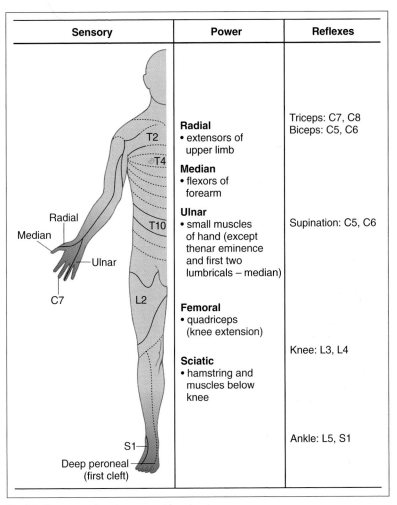	**Radial** • extensors of upper limb **Median** • flexors of forearm **Ulnar** • small muscles of hand (except thenar eminence and first two lumbricals – median) **Femoral** • quadriceps (knee extension) **Sciatic** • hamstring and muscles below knee	Triceps: C7, C8 Biceps: C5, C6 Supination: C5, C6 Knee: L3, L4 Ankle: L5, S1

Fig. 9.3 Sensory and motor nerve aide-mémoire.

(e.g. nerve repair, release of contractures, tendon transfer) has been performed.

EXAMINATION

With the limb under examination and the contralateral limb exposed, inspect for any scars (self-inflicted trauma is a common cause of median nerve damage) and muscle wasting. Is the limb held in a particular position, as in Erb's palsy?

Test the power of the muscle groups in the limb that you are examining, and make comparisons with the contralateral limb. If you suspect a peripheral nerve lesion, pay particular attention to the muscle group(s) supplied by that nerve.

Test for sensation. Use a blunted (but unused) phlebotomy needle to test for pinprick sensation, then cotton wool to test for light touch. The other components of sensation (vibration and temperature) are perhaps more relevant in medical finals. Having established that there is sensory loss, map out the distribution.

Test for limb reflexes using a tendon hammer.

Try to work out whether the neurological deficit suggests a nerve root problem or a peripheral nerve lesion. Fortunately, only a few of the many possible nerve lesions are commonly encountered in exams. Some of these are described below.

Upper brachial plexus lesion***

The condition known as Erb's palsy results from injury to one or more cervical nerve roots, often C5–6.

- Cause: fall on tip of shoulder, obstetric trauma
- Position: arm held internally rotated, forearm pronated
- Sensory deficit: outer aspect of the arm
- Motor deficit: abduction at the shoulder, flexion at the elbow
- Treatment: await recovery; physiotherapy for passive joint movements. Arthrodesis at the shoulder and elbow may be considered.

Lower brachial plexus lesion**

The condition known as Klumpke's palsy typically involves damage to the roots of C8–T1.

- Cause: usually secondary to trauma (e.g. stretching injury of a motorcyclist dragged along the ground), and rarely, as a result of Pancoast's tumour, birth trauma or a cervical rib
- Position: clawhand (plus hyperextension of the MCP joints); more pronounced on the ulnar side of the hand
- Sensory deficit: inner aspect of forearm – three and a half fingers on the ulnar side of the hand
- Motor deficit: weakened flexion and ulnar deviation at the wrist; loss of adduction and abduction of the fingers
- Treatment: await recovery; physiotherapy for passive joint movements. Prognosis is less favourable than with Erb's palsy.

Radial nerve lesion**

- Cause:
  - in the axilla: fractures/dislocations of the humeral head; crutches without hand grips
  - in the radial groove of the humerus: fractures of the humeral shaft; 'Saturday night paralysis' (caused by drunken sleep with the arm over the back of a chair)
- Position: drop wrist may be apparent
- Sensory deficit: proximal division of the nerve leads to loss of sensation over the dorsum of the forearm and dorsum of the first interosseus muscle
- Motor deficit: extension of elbow and wrist (although the long extensors of the fingers are paralysed, the lumbricals can still extend the fingers); extension of the elbow may be saved when the nerve is divided distally
- Treatment: initially, expectant; nerve suture may have a relatively good prognosis, because the radial nerve is predominantly motor.

Median nerve lesion**

See also the section on carpal tunnel syndrome (below).

- Cause:
  - at the elbow: supracondylar humeral fracture
  - at the wrist: lacerations, and occasionally a Colles' fracture; compression as a result of carpal tunnel syndrome
- Position: Simian hand (caused by wasting of the thenar muscles)
- Sensory deficit: anaesthesia over palmar aspects of thumb and index and middle fingers
- Motor deficit: division of the median nerve at the wrist leads to loss of opposition of the thumb; in more proximal lesions there is a weakness of flexion at the wrist, and loss of flexion of the IP (interphalangeal) joint of the thumb
- Treatment: suture of the nerve is required if there is obvious division, but the prognosis is poor because this is a mixed motor and sensory nerve.

Ulnar nerve lesion*

- Cause:
  - at the elbow: fractures, entrapment in the region of the medial epicondyle
  - at the wrist: lacerations

- Position: clawing of the little, ring and middle fingers as a result of wasting of the small muscles of the hand
- Sensory deficit: loss over the little finger and half of the ring finger, anteriorly and posteriorly if the lesion is above the wrist; lesions at the wrist lead only to anterior loss of sensation
- Motor deficit: loss of adduction and abduction of the fingers; with proximal lesions, there is weakness of the long flexors of the little and ring fingers
- Treatment: transposition of the nerve at the elbow, if entrapped.

Sciatic nerve lesion***

- Cause: posterior dislocation of hip, 'intramuscular' injections
- Sensory deficit: total loss of sensation below the knee, except for the inner aspect of the calf
- Motor deficit: complete paralysis below the knee, foot drop, paralysis of the hamstrings.

Lateral popliteal nerve lesion* (Fig. 9.4)

- Cause: fractures of the upper end of the fibula, pressure from plasters, inappropriate positioning on the theatre table
- Sensory deficit: lateral border of the foot
- Motor deficit: dorsiflexion of the foot and dorsiflexion of the great toe (foot drop)

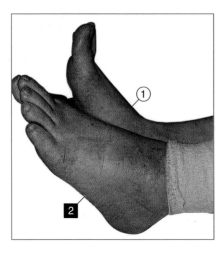

Fig. 9.4 Dropped foot.

① Dorsiflexion of normal foot and great toe

2 Unable to dorsiflex foot or great toe

- Treatment: splinting of the foot in the position of function and awaiting recovery; alternatively, decompression over the head of the fibula may be required.

Carpal tunnel syndrome*

KEY POINTS

- Median nerve distribution of symptoms
- Pressure over carpal tunnel may reproduce symptoms

HISTORY

The presenting symptom of carpal tunnel syndrome is usually pain or paraesthesia, worse at night, in the distribution of the median nerve in the hand and typically in a middle-aged woman. Although usually idiopathic, it may occur in cardiac failure, rheumatoid arthritis, pregnancy, hypothyroidism or acromegaly, or as a complication of a Colles' fracture.

EXAMINATION

With the forearm and hand exposed on both sides, inspection may reveal a scar over the flexor retinaculum on one side (hopefully the asymptomatic, successfully operated-upon side!). Motor loss is unusual. There may be loss of sensation over the palmar aspects of the thumb, index and middle fingers. Pressure on or tapping the carpal tunnel (Tinel's sign) may reproduce the symptoms.

INVESTIGATIONS

Although these findings are commonly quoted in textbooks, nerve conduction studies are required to confirm the diagnosis.

TREATMENT

Treatment is by division of the flexor retinaculum at the wrist, distal to the wrist crease.

Dupuytren's contracture*

Baron Guillaume Dupuytren gained much esteem for treating Napoleon Bonaparte's piles. However, it is a condensation of the palmar fascia that bears his name and Dupuytren's contractures are common short cases in final exams.

HISTORY

You should find out which hand is the dominant hand, and how the contracture interferes with the patient's day-to-day activities. Ask about predisposing causes such as liver disease or recurrent trauma to the palm, remembering that in most patients the contracture has no recognizable cause.

EXAMINATION

On inspection, then palpation, look for a condensation of the palmar fascia into nodules and a band, which may be felt in the palm. As the disease evolves, the fingers (most commonly the little and ring fingers) are drawn into flexion. Thereafter, there is increasing flexion at the MCP and IP joints, resulting in joint contractures.

TREATMENT

Treatment is by excision of the fibrous tissue. Once there is marked deformity of a digit, it is usually difficult to straighten it, and amputation may give the best functional result.

Bursa*

Bursae are, of course, normally present over bony prominences. There are also adventitious bursae, which are newly formed cysts in areas with repeated trauma – the most common is the bursa overlying the first metatarsal in hallux valgus (a bunion). You are most likely to encounter bursae in your short cases, and most commonly a chronic bursitis, occurring in an area subjected to repeated stress.

Hand examination*

Sometimes you will be asked to examine a patient's hands. Remember to look for: nail changes, clubbing, nicotine stains, Heberden's nodes

(DIP), Bouchard's nodes (PIP), gout tophi (periarticular; also on toes, pinnae), rheumatoid changes, bruising, muscle wasting (usually a result of old age, rheumatoid arthritis or cachexia), warts, palmar erythema, Dupuytren's contractures, trigger finger, wasted thenar muscles, T1 root lesion (all the small muscles of the hand are atrophic, with little sensory loss) compared with ulnar nerve palsy (thenar muscles supplied by the median nerve are spared; sensory loss of the ulnar border of the hand), tremor (fine tremor of anxiety, thyrotoxicosis; 'pill-rolling' tremor of Parkinson's disease), function (grip: ask the patient to squeeze two of your fingers; thumb: test strength in opposition to other index finger; test for Froment's sign [grip paper with thumb/index finger]; functional use: holding cup, spoon), sensory loss (index finger tip [median nerve], little finger tip [ulnar nerve], dorsum of first interosseus muscle [radial nerve]) and radial pulse.

Finger clubbing*

Finger clubbing is so common that it usually appears somewhere in finals. You are rarely asked to take a history, but remember the causes if you are. The causes are many, but are best remembered as 'no cause' (idiopathic, familial – the most common category), gastrointestinal (e.g. inflammatory bowel disease such as Crohn's disease, ulcerative colitis; liver cirrhosis), pulmonary (e.g. bronchogenic carcinoma, chronic suppurative lung diseases such as bronchiectasis, fibrosing alveolitis) and heart disease (e.g. congenital cyanotic heart disease, infective endocarditis).

EXAMINATION

On examination, look for the yellow/brown staining of nicotine. Inspect the nails of both hands, commenting on the shape of the nails and terminal phalanges and the nail-bed angle (between the nail and the proximal skin). (Also see Fig. 4.1.)

Gently palpate the nail bed: support the patient's digit with your own two thumbs, then, using your index fingers, elicit fluctuance of the nail bed. You will probably need to demonstrate this on only one digit before you are asked to list some causes of clubbing.

Trigger finger**

Trigger finger (or trigger thumb) is caused by the flexor tendon of the affected digit catching on its sheath at the MCP joint. When the patient straightens the fingers, the affected digit will remain flexed and then suddenly flick out into the extended position. There may be a palpable (sometimes tender) nodule to feel where the tendon catches.

Mallet finger***

A mallet finger results from the rupture of the long extensor tendon where it inserts into the distal phalange, producing a typical deformity (see Fig. 9.2).

THE BACK

The back has been included in this chapter because patients with nerve root compression resulting from back problems may present with lower limb symptoms in surgical finals. In such a case you will be expected to differentiate between the compression of a nerve root and a specific peripheral nerve lesion. The most common presentation of pathology in the back is pain, usually in the lumbar region.

HISTORY

If you are presented with a patient with back problems, establish their age. Disc problems are most common in the age range 30–45 years, after which there is a progressive increase in the incidence of osteoarthritis. In older patients, metastatic carcinoma should be considered. Ask particularly about the onset, site, radiation, exacerbating factors, relieving factors and severity of any pain, which may lead you quickly to the diagnosis.

An acute disc prolapse will often occur when the patient has lifted something heavy or sneezed, and is associated with severe pain and 'locking' of the back. The pain may well shoot down the patient's leg in the distribution of L5 or S1 nerve roots (from the buttock to distal to the knee). Disc pain may have a more chronic onset and present first with nerve root irritation. Similarly, other causes of back pain may have an insidious onset (e.g. metastatic disease, osteoarthritis and spondylolisthesis). In addition to asking about back pain and radiation of the pain, find out about the impact of the symptoms on the patient's lifestyle. Ask particularly about the patient's work, and whether there is any question of industrial injury or compensation claims. You must not forget to enquire about related medical problems, such as osteoarthritis in other joints, the possibility of metastatic cancer (often lung, breast or prostate) or referred to the back from other sites, such as the pancreas. Finally remember that back pain may be a symptom of intra–abdominal pathology, i.e. an aortic aneurysm or a pancreatic carcinoma.

EXAMINATION

Your system for examining the back should follow the same pattern as that established for other orthopaedic problems:

- look
- feel
- move.

After this, you should conduct a full neurological examination, looking for signs of nerve root compression.

Look

It is helpful to watch a patient's gait and examine the spinal curvature with the patient wearing a minimum of underclothes, so that you can observe movements of the spine. Look particularly for the typical 'half-shut knife' position of someone leaning forward with a partially flexed, painful back. There may be flattening of the normal lumbar lordosis as a result of erector spinae spasm, which if more marked on one side may lead to a scoliosis. Comment also on any visible 'steps' or marked kyphosis that may have resulted from vertebral collapse.

Feel

Ask whether the patient has any tenderness before you palpate the spine. Localized tenderness may occur over an area of pathology, and may identify the level of a lesion. Unfortunately, it will not differentiate between different types of lesion affecting the back, e.g. crush fractures, metastatic disease or disc problems. You may be able to feel a specific 'step' in cases of spondylolisthesis, or a localized kyphosis in a patient with vertebral collapse.

Move

Test for flexion and extension, but watch to see that the back is moving: a patient with ankylosing spondylitis, when asked to touch the toes, may bend forwards at the hips even though the back is completely fused. Lateral flexion to the left and right should be determined, again watching to ensure that this is not achieved by tilting the pelvis. Holding the pelvis steady, assess rotation to the left and right. Flexion, extension, lateral flexion and rotation can be tested for the cervical, thoracic and lumbar spine, recognizing that the range of each type of movement will be different in each part of the spine.

With the patient lying supine, perform the straight leg raise: with the knee fully extended, gently elevate the leg – there will be limitation of straight leg raising if there is nerve root irritation. Dorsiflexion of the foot or pressure over the popliteal fossa will exacerbate sciatic nerve pain radiating from the lumbar spine to distal to the knee. Movement at the hip may be free, and often there is a full range of hip flexion provided that the knee is flexed. The femoral stretch test (with the patient lying prone and the hip passively extended) is not very likely to be required of you in the exam.

Neurological examination

If you suspect vertebral collapse or a prolapsed disc it is essential to assess the patient's neurological status (see Fig. 9.3). This will involve the assessment of:

- power (graded 0–5, see page 231)
- sensation (to pinprick and touch as a basic minimum)
- reflexes (in the affected limbs)

and comparing the findings with your assessment of the contralateral limb.

TYPICAL CASES

Lumbar disc prolapse**

This is the most common type of disc prolapse, and the one most likely to be encountered in exams.

HISTORY

Take a history as outlined above, asking particularly about the patient's job, the symptoms of pain (which should be differentiated from pain caused by peripheral vascular disease), and the limitations they impose on everyday activities such as sitting and bending (e.g. putting on socks).

Paraesthesia or numbness may also be symptoms of disc prolapse or nerve compression, and establishing which parts of the limb have altered sensation will often guide you to the nerve roots involved. Loss of control of the bladder or bowel is unlikely to be present in a patient used in surgical finals, but you should still ask about these symptoms, because they imply a surgical emergency. Ask what analgesia or other relieving tactics (such as lying on the floor) have been tried.

EXAMINATION

The patient with an acute disc prolapse will hold the back in a slightly flexed position, and you will see loss of the normal lordosis and marked erector spinae spasm.

It is likely that there will be tenderness over the relevant vertebral body, and also over the tense erector spinae muscles.

The most common disc prolapses are L4–5 (catching the L5 nerve root) and L5–S1 (affecting the S1 nerve root). In both cases there is limitation of straight leg raising. Lesions affecting L5 will cause weakness of dorsiflexion of the ankle and the great toe, and sensory loss over the dorsum of the foot. The ankle jerk will be present. In contrast, S1 lesions will result in loss of the ankle jerk, weakness of plantar flexion of the ankle and toes, and anaesthesia along the outer aspect of the foot. Rarely, prolapse of a higher disc may affect the L4 nerve root, resulting in weakness of the quadriceps and loss of the knee-jerk reflex. In this case, stretching the femoral nerve is painful. This is done by asking the patient to lie on his or her front and gently extend the hip with the knee flexed.

Occasionally, a disc prolapse will protrude centrally, compressing the spinal cord. This will lead to bilateral symptoms, loss of anal sphincter control and bladder paresis. It is very unlikely that you will see such a patient in the exam, because this is a surgical emergency, but you may be asked about it. Cervical disc lesions are much less common than lumbar disc problems, and neurological sequelae are unusual because of the comparatively large vertebral foramen in the cervical region.

INVESTIGATION

The differential diagnosis of lumbar disc prolapse includes osteoarthritis, spondylolisthesis, metastatic tumours, and primary and secondary spinal tumours. You should therefore ask for blood biochemistry including urea, electrolytes, calcium, phosphate, and prostate-specific antigen (PSA – a marker of prostate cancer), and for the ESR.

A plain radiograph may not show any specific lesion, but may help to exclude part of the differential diagnosis. Prolapse of a disc through the endplate into the vertebral body may result in the radiological appearance of Schmorl's node. Other radiological signs may include narrowing of disc spaces and secondary osteoarthritic changes. If surgery is contemplated, the level of the disc prolapse should be identified from CT or MRI. If metastatic disease is suspected, but not demonstrated on plain radiographs, a bone scan may be informative and may demonstrate the cause of the symptoms.

MANAGEMENT

Most disc prolapses will resolve with conservative measures: bed rest and certainly the avoidance of any heavy lifting or vigorous activity until the pain subsides. Analgesia and antispasmodics can give great relief. In cases that either fail to settle or recur, surgery should be considered. An absolute and urgent indication for surgery is the development of bladder paralysis from a central disc prolapse. Progressive muscle weakness would also indicate the need for decompression. Microdiscectomy or hemilaminectomy should be performed in order to remove the prolapsed disc material.

Secondary tumour deposits in the vertebrae**

These are relatively common compared with primary spinal tumours as a cause of back pain, and may cause vertebral collapse and cord compression.

HISTORY

The patient may give you a history of a previous carcinoma, or alternatively this may be the first sign of a carcinoma (particularly in the case of prostatic carcinoma or multiple myeloma). The presentation may simply be back pain, or alternatively progressive vertebral collapse may lead to neurological symptoms such as pain in the girdle region and progressive weakness (usually of the lower limbs).

EXAMINATION

There may be little to see and only localized tenderness on examination of the back. Alternatively, you may see signs of vertebral collapse, including kyphosis or scoliosis. If there is cord compression the patient, if mobile, will have a broad-based gait. There may be signs of increased muscle tone and a spastic paresis in the lower limbs (typical of an upper motor neuron paralysis). Remember to look also for signs of the primary tumour, the most common being breast, prostate, bronchus, kidney and thyroid.

INVESTIGATION

Investigations should be performed in order to determine the site of the primary tumour. With regard to the bony lesion, clinical biochemistry may show elevated calcium and phosphate together with elevated alkaline phosphatase, but these are non-specific indicators of bone activity.

Plain radiographs may demonstrate either sclerotic lesions (particularly in prostatic carcinoma and breast cancer) or lytic lesions (Fig. 9.5), but may also be normal in the case of early lesions. A bone scan using radioisotopes will show an area of increased uptake corresponding to metastatic bone lesions (Fig, 9.6), but this finding is non-specific and

Fig. 9.5 Radiograph of the pelvis and femoral shafts with lytic lesions in the right neck and shaft of the femur.

Fig. 9.6 Isotope bone scan of the same patient as Fig. 9.5, showing bone metastases in the right femoral shaft and pelvis.

should be regarded as showing metastatic tumour only if associated with normal radiographs or typical lesions of bony secondaries (rather than benign changes such as those of arthritis). If there are signs of cord compression, the level and extent of this should be delineated by means of CT or MRI.

MANAGEMENT

Conservative measures (such as the use of a walking stick) and analgesia may provide considerable relief. Rehydration (if bone metastases have caused hypercalcaemia) and treatment of the hypercalcaemia with bisphosphonates can be very effective.

Treatment of the primary tumour may also be effective in the treatment of the bony disease (e.g. tamoxifen in breast cancer or orchidectomy [surgical or chemical] in prostatic cancer). Localized radiotherapy is often successful in the control of pain caused by the tumour. In cases where there is cord compression, it may be necessary to consider surgical decompression: when there is vertebral collapse, this will involve initial stabilization of the spine.

KEY QUESTIONS

1. What is the basic examination scheme for orthopaedic patients?
2. How would you describe a fracture?
3. In general terms, how would you treat a patient with a fracture?
4. What is the typical deformity of a Colles' fracture and how is this fracture caused?
5. Which systems may be involved in rheumatoid arthritis?
6. How would you examine the hip?
7. How would you classify muscle power?
8. What are the features of an ulnar nerve palsy?
9. What are the key features of:
   - Dupuytren's contracture?
   - Finger clubbing?
10. How would you differentiate between a ganglion and a sebaceous cyst?
11. What features of disease might you see on a patient's hands?
12. What are the differences between the neurological findings in a lateral peroneal nerve lesion and a prolapse of the L5–S1 intervertebral disc?
13. Answer the following as true or false:
    - Prolapsed cervical discs commonly cause neurological symptoms.
    - Lumbar disc prolapse is a condition of elderly people.
    - Carpal tunnel syndrome leads to wasting of the interosseous muscles.
    - The radial nerve is commonly damaged in Colles' fractures.
    - The sciatic nerve is in danger after dislocation of the hip.
    - Rheumatoid arthritis usually affects the DIP joints.
    - The ankle jerk reflex is absent in an L5–S1 disc prolapse.
    - Bony metastases may not be apparent on plain radiographs

10

Other useful topics

There are some topics that can come up in the clinical parts or the oral parts of surgical finals, and are usually related to a patient whom you have been asked to examine.

TRAUMA AND RESUSCITATION

Injury can be described as blunt injury, penetrating (knife/firearms) injury or blast injury. The history will give hints as to the likely patterns of injury. Whatever the type of injury, the ABC of trauma resuscitation forms the basis of how to resuscitate a patient following trauma, in any emergency situation including surgical finals:

- A for **a**irway, with cervical spine control
- B for **b**reathing
- C for **c**irculation.

A – airway

Clear and then maintain the airway (while keeping the cervical spine controlled in the case of trauma patients):

- Clear obstruction of the airway by foreign bodies/tongue
- Maintain the airway by chin lift/jaw thrust
- Insert an oropharyngeal airway/cuffed endotracheal tube, or use cricoid needle/cricothyroidotomy if required.

B – breathing

Ensure that the patient is breathing:

- Assist breathing if necessary
- Supply high-flow oxygen if necessary
- Beware (tension) pneumothorax and flail segments.

C – circulation

Control bleeding and maintain circulating blood volume:

- Control external bleeding with pressure
- Control internal bleeding if possible (e.g. splint fractures)
- Restore circulating blood volume (using crystalloids and matched (preferably) or blood group O rhesus-negative blood), via two large-bore venous cannulae (use pulse and urine output as measures of circulating blood volume).

D – conduct survey

Perform survey from head to toe of fully exposed patient, including all orifices.

HEAD INJURY (also see page 70, Fig. 3.18)

- Prevent secondary brain injury caused by hypoxia, hypercapnia, hypotension, intracranial bleeding
- Beware extradural haematoma (usually resulting from injury of the middle meningeal vessels) – classically presents with a transient loss of consciousness, a lucid interval, then deterioration of the conscious level
- Beware facial/mandibular fractures, causing airway impairment and/or blood loss.

CHEST INJURY

- Beware tension pneumothorax/haemothorax
- Beware rib fractures
- Beware cardiac injury
- Beware penetrating injuries.

ABDOMINAL INJURY

- Beware occult intra-abdominal bleeding (a diagnostic peritoneal lavage may be needed)
- Perform anal and rectal examination
- Test urine for blood
- Catheterize if no urethral or perineal injury
- Insert nasogastric tube.

EXTREMITY INJURIES

- Splint injured limbs, to reduce pain and blood loss
- Control bleeding from vascular injuries
- Beware compartment syndrome
- Clean, débride and explore wounds
- Ensure anti-tetanus prophylaxis.

RADIOLOGY

You may well be asked to look at and comment on a radiograph as part of a long or a short case or in a viva. You will not be expected to be an expert radiologist but you will be expected to approach a radiograph sensibly, demonstrate a methodical approach to interpreting the films, and detect abnormalities. What are being tested are your approach and your powers of observation. You may be given a short history before you are asked to look at a radiograph, or you may be shown a film from your long or short case. The term 'X-ray' may be used in everyday speech, but is considered bad slang in exams.

There are guidelines that make the interpretation of radiographs (of whatever type) easier, especially in the heat of an exam when all knowledge and reason seem to desert you:

1. Always view the film or films on a well-lit viewing box.
2. Check that the film is the right way up, and oriented correctly with the 'R' marker on what would be the patient's right-hand side if you were standing talking to him or her. If there are several films (e.g. a barium enema series), the examiner will usually choose one for you.
3. Check the patient's name and date of birth if they are visible.
4. Avoid touching the radiograph thereafter (lots of sweaty fingers during an exam start to irritate the examiners, because the fingers often mark the films). Ask if you want to touch the film.
5. Decide what type of film you are examining: e.g. state to the examiner 'This is a CT scan of the abdomen through the liver' (Fig. 10.1). This makes you sound confident, avoids embarrassing silences and gives you time to think!
6. Stand back and get an overall impression. Is there a gross abnormality that strikes you immediately?
7. Now study the radiograph systematically: keep talking, stating what you are looking for even if there is no abnormality present.

Fig. 10.1 Cross-sectional CT scan through the liver demonstrating multiple liver metastases and a gastric mass.

8. As you spot abnormalities, describe them: 'There are multiple lesions in the liver.'
9. Look for a second abnormality, or even more than two: 'There is a thickening of the lesser curve of the stomach with a fungating mass in the lumen.'
10. Take a further look to ensure that you haven't missed anything that now seems obvious.
11. Summarize what you see, e.g. 'This is a cross-sectional CT through the liver showing multiple liver metastases and a gastric mass.'

The aim of this approach to radiographs is to give you a routine, which allows you to demonstrate a systematic way of examining the film, so that you can not only describe the obvious but (with luck) pick up more subtle features that you might otherwise miss. The best way to establish this routine is to practise with a fellow student, a tutor or (preferably) a radiologist, not once but many times, using different films showing different abnormalities.

FLUID BALANCE/NUTRITION

Some patients in surgical finals may have a drip attached, or may be receiving parenteral nutrition.

Fluid/electrolyte balance

The topic of fluid and electrolyte balance can give you sleepless nights, trying to remember exact values, and the many upset states that are possible in patients. The essential concept to remember is that what is lost must be replaced. Working out the types of fluid/ electrolytes lost, and the sites of loss, gives you a clue to the patient's requirements. A normal adult's basic daily needs are:

- Sodium: 70–80 mmol (one 500 ml bag of 0.9% saline)
- Potassium: 60 mmol (falling to 20 mmol first postoperative day)
- Water: 1000 ml (minimum).

The possible routes, and the corresponding extents, of fluid losses and gains are summarized in Table 10.1. Those represented by a '?' are highly variable.

Table 10.1 Fluid balance

	Losses (ml/day)		Gains (ml/day)
Normal			
Urine	1500	Endogenous water	300
Insensible			
– breathing	700		
– sweat	200		
Faeces	200		
Possible			
Gastric (nasogastric tube/vomit)	2500	Oral	?
Bile duct (via T tube)	1500	Intravenous	?
Pancreatic	1000	Intravenous additives	?
Small bowel fistula	3000	Central line	?
Diarrhoea	15 000		
Sequestration			
– to wound site	500		
– from drains	?		
– into chest cavity	?		
– peritoneum (ascites)	?		

Nutrition

The normal daily nutritional requirements of a 70 kg man are:

- 9–15 g nitrogen
- 2000–3000 kcal (including 200 kcal of non-protein energy per g nitrogen, of which 60–80 kcal should be provided by fat)
- 2–3 l fluid
- Electrolytes (including 70 mmol sodium and 60 mmol potassium)
- Trace elements, minerals and vitamins.

Nutrition can be given via the gastrointestinal tract (the enteral route – by mouth or tube [nasogastric, nasoduodenal, gastrostomy or jejunostomy]), or intravenously as parenteral nutrition (via a peripheral or central vein).

Oral/enteral nutrition can be in the form of normal food, fluid feed or elemental diet. Complications of the enteral route include nausea, vomiting, bloating and diarrhoea, and wound problems at the insertion site of the feeding tube (in the case of gastrostomy/jejunostomy).

Complications of parenteral nutrition include those of catheter insertion (e.g. haematoma, pneumothorax, air embolus), thrombophlebitis (especially with peripheral lines), cardiac dysrhythmias (resulting from the tip of the line) and infection (at the skin entry site or of the catheter); infection may in turn result in septicaemia and metabolic disturbance (e.g. hyperosmolar syndrome, electrolyte imbalance, abnormal liver function, deficiency syndromes).

PREOPERATIVE INVESTIGATIONS

Preparation of a patient for surgery is one of the most common tasks for recently qualified doctors – hence it is often a topic in surgical finals.

Cardiac disease, respiratory conditions and fluid/electrolyte disturbance (see above) are key areas. Although some investigations may be considered essential in all patients undergoing general anaesthesia (e.g. haemoglobin), patients aged >45 years and patients with symptoms of cardiorespiratory disease require more rigorous investigations selected from the following list.

Investigations

- Urinary testing for glucose in people with diabetes, proteins in renal disease

- Haematology may show anaemia (microcytic/macrocytic) as an exacerbating factor in cardiorespiratory symptoms
- Prothrombin time ratio or international normalised ratio for control of warfarin
- Biochemistry (ureas, sodium, potassium) may confirm electrolyte disturbances, which can precipitate or worsen cardiac dysrhythmias
- Arterial blood gas for arterial P_{O_2}, P_{CO_2} and acid–base balance may confirm the presence of hypoxia or hypercapnia and/or compensatory changes in metabolic or respiratory acidosis or alkalosis
- Blood transfusion: group and save, crossmatch (number of units depends on likely extent of surgery)
- Chest PA (posteroanterior) radiograph
- A 12-lead ECG may be used to assess cardiac rate and rhythm and signs of current or previous myocardial damage
- A treadmill/stress ECG and/or 24-hour monitoring tape may elicit signs of myocardial disease
- Echocardiography can be used to examine the structure and function of the heart muscle, heart valves and blood flow
- Spirometry may be used to measure the FEV_1 (forced expiratory volume in 1 s) FVC (forced vital capacity), FEV_1/FVC ratio and more complex measures of respiratory function.

ANALGESIA

Although this subject is covered fully in textbooks on anaesthesia, analgesia is a favourite topic when discussing postoperative patient management, perhaps as part of a long case. You should be able to discuss the following methods and their uses (Table 10.2):

Table 10.2 Analgesia

Local analgesia	Systemic analgesia
Skin gel:	Paracetamol
– local anaesthetic	NSAIDs
– non-steroidal anti-inflammatory drug (NSAID)	Opiates:
Injected local anaesthetic:	– dihydrocodeine
– lidocaine (short-acting)	– pethidine
– bupivicaine (long-acting)	– morphine
Regional nerve blockade:	
– local nerves (just as at the dentist!)	
– regional caudal block	
– epidural	

The methods of delivery of analgesia include oral (tablet/sublingual/liquid), per rectum (suppository), intermittent injections, infusion and patient-controlled analgesia (PCA). Antiemetics can be added to these.

POSTOPERATIVE COMPLICATIONS

Postoperative complications, such as those listed, can occur after any operation and fall into two categories, local to and distant to the site of surgery (Table 10.3).

Table 10.3 Postoperative complications	
Distant to site of surgery	**At site of surgery**
Pulmonary atelectasis	Haemorrhage
Pneumonia	Nerve damage
Fluid overload	Wound infection
Phlebitis	Abscess
DVT/pulmonary embolus	Ileus
Urinary tract infection	Wound dehiscence
Central line sepsis	Anastomotic leakage
Transfusion reactions	Fistula
Renal failure	
Pressure sores	

DEEP VENOUS THROMBOSIS (DVT)

Development

DVT develops during/after 30% of surgical operations. The three main aetiological factors are venous stasis, enhanced coagulation and intimal damage (Virchow's triad). The many risk factors include: age > 40 years, malignancy, obesity, abdominal surgery, hip/knee replacement surgery, previous DVT or embolus, and the oral contraceptive pill.

Prevention is assisted by: subcutaneous low-dose heparin started preoperatively (e.g. 5000 U twice daily), graduated compression stockings, early mobilization, intermittent pneumatic compression boots intraoperatively and Dextran 70.

Detection

Detection of DVT depends on: clinical suspicion (although clinical diagnosis of a warm, swollen, tender calf is notoriously unreliable), bilateral ascending venography and Doppler ultrasonography.

Pulmonary embolism may be revealed by a ventilation–perfusion scan. Chest radiographs and an ECG are likely to be more useful for excluding other causes of chest symptoms than in the diagnosis of pulmonary embolism.

Treatment

- For calf vein thrombosis alone: graduated compression stockings and mobilize (low risk of embolism)
- If iliofemoral segment involved: bed rest and anticoagulation with heparin for 7–10 days, then oral warfarin for 3–6 months
- If high risk of embolism, particularly if non-occlusive: thrombolytic therapy or thrombectomy
- For recurrent embolism not controlled by other means, consider insertion of a vena caval filter.

SURGICAL TUBES/DRAINS

In surgical finals, it is useful to decide what a tube attached to the patient may be there for – this may give you helpful information for working out the diagnosis and treatment.

Tubes attached to patients can be either entry tubes (allow something into the body) or exit tubes (let things leave). They can be categorized by function:

- Vascular access:
  - intravenous line
  - central venous line (fluids/feed/chemotherapy)
  - arterial line (sampling blood/measuring pressures)
  - AV (arteriovenous) fistula (for dialysis)
- Respiratory access:
  - endotracheal tube
  - tracheostomy
- Gastrointestinal access:
  - nasogastric tube (free drainage, continuous/intermittent suction)
  - nasoduodenal tube (feeding)
  - gastrostomy tube (feeding/drainage)
  - jejunostomy tube (feeding)
  - biliary drainage tube (e.g. T-tube)
- Body cavity access:
  - chest drain
  - abdominal drain (suction/free drainage/dialysis tube).

What comes out of the drain can give you a hint as to where the tube is. Nasogastric aspirates may be: opalescent, likened to ginger beer (pure gastric); golden (bile stained); green (from the small bowel); or faeculent (brown, foul smelling, from the lower small bowel). Abdominal drains may produce blood, serous fluid, bile or bowel content.

WOUND HEALING

The healing of soft tissue wounds takes 4–5 days on the face and 10–14 days on the trunk and limbs to gain sufficient strength to enable removal of the sutures without disruption to the wound. Further strengthening occurs over about 6 months.

Healing can be by first intention (close and accurate apposition of incised wounds), second intention (defect fills in with granulation tissue and scar contraction shrinks wound size) or third intention (a wound healing by secondary intention is surgically sutured to achieve apposition). Hypertrophic scars (exaggerated normal healing) are raised, red and firm, and may resolve over time. In contrast, keloid scars continue to worsen and enlarge after 6 months.

Factors (particularly adverse factors) affecting wound healing (Table 10.4) can be divided into general factors and local factors, either of which may occur after any operation or specific to a particular operation.

Table 10.4 Factors influency wound healing

General factors	Local factors
Age	Site
Jaundice	Tissue damage
Anaemia	Ischaemia
Hypoxia	Bacterial contamination
Steroids	Infection
Immunosuppression	Radiotherapy
Diabetes	Foreign material
Malnutrition	Failure of apposition

For example, wound healing might fail in an elderly patient with diabetes (general factors) with a pretibial laceration (site, tissue damage, ischaemia).

WOUND INFECTION

Wounds can be classed as clean (wound contamination not expected, infection rate <1%, e.g. thyroidectomy), clean contaminated (no frank infection but significant risk of infection, although should be <5%, e.g. cholecystectomy) or contaminated (dirty operations, e.g. surgery for perforated colon).

Prevention of infection should include preoperative skin cleaning (patient's skin and surgeon's hands), reduction in potential contamination (e.g. clearing the colon of faeces before a sigmoid resection), antibiotic prophylaxis against likely contaminating organisms (which may depend on the site, e.g. different for hip replacement and colonic surgery) and use of sterile equipment.

Signs of wound infection (at 3–4 days postoperatively) include the features of inflammation (hot, red, swollen, tender, loss of function), discharge from the wound, pyrexia and leukocytosis, and (with severe infection) bacteraemia, septicaemia and even death. In contrast, wound haematomas occur earlier (usually with few systemic signs, although they may predispose to infection), and deep wound dehiscence occurs later (at 7–10 days, usually accompanied by a profuse serous discharge, followed by the abdominal organs emerging through the wound). However, wound infection may become apparent some time (even years) after surgery, e.g. related to a non-absorbable abdominal suture or an orthopaedic prosthesis.

Index